ONE MORE PUFF

The Truth Behind Nicotine's Grip

Dr. Leelamohan PVR

AF516703

BlueRose ONE.com
Stories Matter
NewDelhi • London

BLUEROSE PUBLISHERS
India | U.K.

For permissions requests or inquiries regarding this publication, please contact:

BLUEROSE PUBLISHERS
www.BlueRoseONE.com
info@bluerosepublishers.com
+91 8882 898 898
+4407342408967

ISBN: 978-93-7310-447-8

Cover design: Yash Singhal
Typesetting: Namrata Saini

First Edition: October 2025

Dedication

This book is dedicated to all my patients,

my friends,

my supporters,

my parents –

Parthasarathy and **Ramadevi,**

and every beautiful soul in my life who lights up my path with love and encouragement.

May this work serve to educate, inspire, and empower every reader toward a healthier, smoke-free life.

Preface

We often remember the first cigarette—not because it was pleasant, but because of what followed. For some, it started as an act of rebellion. For others, it was curiosity, peer pressure, or simply a way to cope with stress. But very few realize, in that first puff, they were unknowingly inviting a lifelong guest into their body—nicotine—a guest that promises comfort but demands control.

As a doctor, I've seen what nicotine can do—not just to lungs and hearts, but to lives, families, careers, and futures. Over the years, I've treated patients who came in for a "mild cough" only to discover something far more serious. I've met individuals who could not go a single morning without a cigarette—and others who believed vaping was their safe escape, not knowing the truth.

This book is my attempt to bridge the gap between science and real life—to take what we know in medical literature and translate it into something everyone can understand. Whether you're a smoker, an ex-smoker, a concerned family member, or a curious reader, this book is for you.

You will learn about how nicotine hijacks the brain, how addiction forms, how tobacco traveled across continents, how it's been celebrated, sold, and embedded into our culture. But more importantly, this book will walk you through why it's so hard to quit, and why it's still absolutely possible.

This is not a book of judgment. It is a book of awareness, hope, and empowerment. Smoking is not a weakness; it is an addiction. And addiction, like any illness, deserves understanding—and treatment.

As you turn these pages, I invite you to read with curiosity, compassion, and courage. If it makes you reflect, share, or help even one person on their journey toward freedom, then this book will have done its job.

Thank you for giving it your time—and perhaps, a little piece of your truth.

Dr. Leelamohan PVR

MBBS, MD

Consultant Physician & Diabetologist

Padithem Health Care, Bangalore

Acknowledgement

I express my heartfelt gratitude to all the wonderful people who have supported me throughout this journey.

First and foremost, I sincerely thank my patients, who inspire me every day with their resilience and trust. Their experiences and stories motivated me to write this book, aiming to create awareness and help people make informed decisions about their health.

I am deeply grateful to my friends and well-wishers who encouraged me to take this step and stood by me through every stage of this process. Your constant support, feedback, and belief in my vision were invaluable.

Special thanks to my parents, my loving father **Parthasarathy** and my caring mother **Ramadevi**, whose unconditional love, wisdom, and blessings shaped the person I am today.

Finally, I dedicate this work to all the beautiful people in my life—those who bring light, kindness, and inspiration every single day. Thank you for making this possible.

Contents

Chapter – 1
NICOTIANA

Do you remember your first nicotine hit? The holy ritual of lighting up a cigarette, whiffing a puff, the little strain in the throat during inhalation, and the unremarkable fleeting feeling which, in an instant, soothes your brain.

The addiction to nicotine, its charisma, is as ancient as human curiosity.

Nicotine is infamous for causing an intoxicated hit. It comes from the tobacco plant which is actually indigenous to the Americas. However, its multi-purpose and high-utility brought it fame. The plant is now known in far corners of the world for its healing properties, but mainly for its intoxicating nature.

If we dig into history, it was around 8000 years ago that tobacco was first cultivated near the Andes region, which is in present day Peru. After thousands of years of history and a long journey with traders from one country to another, the plant reached the Indian subcontinent during the 1600s. For a long time, the natives of the Americas made use of the available wild species like *nicotiana rustica* and *nicotiana tabacum*. But around 3000 BCE, the cultivation began first in Mesoamerica and the Caribbean, consisting of present day Mexico, El Salvador, Costa Rica, and Guatemala. The primitives held it in high regard for its spiritual relevance, making it part of ceremonies. They believed the smoke to be mystical, possessing powers which could take them to heaven. Historically, it was used to attend to various physical ailments and helped with pain alleviation, respiratory issues and more. Over time, its various uses ingrained it deeply in American history.

With continued efforts and experiments, various ways of consumption were developed. People loved chewing the leaves, inhaling the smoke through pipes, and snuffing the powdered leaves. It became part of entertainment and was widely consumed in various regions in North and South America. Soon the Europeans became familiar with the plant as more travellers came to the Americas. They cherished learning its uses and took it back to their homes. This is how Christopher Columbus learned about the wonders of smoking tobacco from the Taino tribe on his excursion. The Tainos lived in Caribbean regions, sustaining themselves by fishing and farming. They made the most of the resources from the sea like shells and fishes . Christopher, in his accounts, talked about their kindness and highlighted the hearty trade they shared.

Through trade, tobacco crossed seas and reached different lands of Europe, mainly with the Spanish explorers. People first felt sceptical of the smoke, mistaking it for witchcraft, but slowly, when its medicinal properties were revealed, its acceptance grew. The popular folklore is that King James I of England was tremendously against smoking tobacco. He circulated a pamphlet titled "A Counterblast to Tobacco" explaining its gruesome nature and urging citizens to give up on its usage. However, soon, the clouds of doubts cleared. Jean Nicot de Villemain was a French diplomat who, on a mission to Portugal, sent the plant's seed to The Queen mother Catherine de Medici. This way, he became the first to introduce tobacco in France in 1560, explaining to people its medical benefits. The plant worked so effectively that it was renamed *Nicotiana* in his honor. King Francis II promoted its use and people from across the world become curious to try it. Soon, with Portuguese traders, the plant travelled to Asia and Africa, entering the Indian subcontinent.

NEXT DESTINATION- INDIA!

The then emperor of India, Akbar, graciously welcomed the traders who brought with them the tobacco plant in India. Within a short span of time, its craze spread everywhere. It became so popular that to get the situation under control, Akbar's successor Jahangir had to put a ban on it in 1617. But the seeds had been sown. The first tobacco plant had already been established by then in 1613 in Gujarat, the surplus from which was exported to Pegu and Arakan.

Nicotine was yet to undergo the standard scientific research and studied thoroughly. Even though it was known worldwide, it was only in 1843 that its molecular formula was coded. The curiosity which first grippled the minds was more to do with what is it that with just one puff the mind and mood instantly alters, changing our perspective, giving one the lordly strength to face anxieties again?

The history of "a hit" goes long back. In India, the Mughals lauded the tobacco filled hookah pipes. They were adorned in the courts and were part of all lavish celebrations and festivities. The legacy of tobacco was passed down from hookah pipes to a roll of cigarette during the British Raj. A symbol of sophistication, superior status, a sign of luxury, tobacco filled in hookahs, and later in cigarettes was glorified by the emperors and later the British colonels. This produced a heavy demand for tobacco in the form of cigars and bidis during the British times. The demand eventually led to the expansion in the cultivation of tobacco. In Andhra Pradesh, Gujarat, and Assam, huge production units were established to meet the growing taste for tobacco consumption. Over time, new variants of consumption emerged. One of the most popular was *bidi*, which, because of its cheap rates, was preferred by the working class. Even in 21st century modern India, labourers can often be seen in a nook, lighting a bidi roll during breaks. The craze of tobacco is wild that popular and hit bollywood songs are also named after it to pull in audiences.

WHAT IS HAPPENING TODAY?

When India gained independence from the British Raj, it continued the production of tobacco. The demand did not slow down. With the coming of industrialisation, and India entering into a more free economy, we saw the establishments of huge companies like Indian Tobacco Company, popularly known as ITC. In later chapters, we will see how tobacco use has been revolutionised in the modern scientific society.

Mid 20th century favoured easy availability of tobacco, cheap prices, and a wide variety of flavors. This contributed to the high rate of growing consumers. It was the time when Indian society went through many cultural changes. There was a push towards education bringing a change in the young minds. The liberal youth, believers of modernity, smoked cigarettes to cherish their newfound freedom in adulthood. The cigarettes grew in popularity, sidelining the traditional way of inhalation. But still, in pubs today one can enjoy the royalty of the hookah.

Over centuries, tobacco has become a part of the national economy and our day to day lives. The medium of consumption has changed with time but its still widely popular. At present, India accounts for 9 percent of the total global production of tobacco employing 45.7 million people. It is a well and thriving business yielding huge profits for the economy and generating employment. As per a report from the ICAR- Central Tobacco Research Institution, tobacco industry contributes 4,400 crores to the foreign exchange. Thus, the power of a puff is undeniable. It has a significant role in maintaining the GDP of the country.

The journey of tobacco is ingrained in a large socio-cultural and economic context. But let's face the bitter truth - it takes more than it gives. India loses 1 percent of its GDP every year because of tobacco deaths. If we talk in terms of numbers, it is close to 1.35 million early deaths every year.

What now seems like a short *sutta* break is actually slow death in the long term. It is disguised as a quick fix to alleviate stress or boost up concentration, but in reality, every puff is slowly degrading your body. If you think it only damages your lungs, giving rise to respiratory illness, you might not be completely aware of the larger picture which is more grave. The journey begins in the brain causing both, physiological and psychological complications. First it is labored breathing while taking staircases, then issues with concentration and later with memory and finally, cognitive damage. This book is an attempt to explain how Nicotine impacts your brain leaving an addictive imprint which can prove to be fatal.

What is so sparkly about a cigarette that keeps pulling people?

The magic of the tobacco laden cigarette roll is actually in the nicotine present in it. People smoke tobacco for an instant feeling of relaxation, a sense of pleasure which is often associated with a feeling of accomplishment. But what is Nicotine - just an intoxicant, hijacking our brain?

For a better understanding of how nicotine works let's break it down. Technically speaking, Nicotine (C6H14N2) is a naturally occurring alkaloid which is found most in tobacco plants. Tobacco belongs to the *Solanaceae* family, also known as the nightshade family along with eggplants, tomato, and peppers. These vegetables also have a minute amount of nicotine, but in the tobacco plant, the concentration is very high. That's why there is no tomato addiction.

Nicotine is made of two rings - *Pyridine* and *Pyrrolidine*. These rings are joined by a single bond which carries all the functional activities. They are like pair of scissors helping nicotine bond with the n*icotinic acetylcholine receptors* found in the human central nervous system. It has many subtypes out of which the a4b2* makes it highly sensitive to nicotine.

WHO IS MR.NICOTINE?

You can have a look at the physical state of nicotine to ease your curiosity. It is a yellowish liquid which can turn brown when exposed to air by the simple process of oxidation. You can taste and smell it but may not like it, since it has a bitter taste and is also a toxin. It has high solubility in water and alcohol, making it possible to get easily absorbed in the human body. When reacted with acids, it forms salts. These are easily water soluble and hence used in e-cigarettes for better experience. Its other features like its high lipophilicity, meaning its ability to dissolve in oils, lipids and fats, enables it to cross the blood brain barrier, allowing it a quick entry inside your brain. It is volatile, making it easy to light and inhale through smoking and vaping. Needless to say, it is also known for its toxicity for human consumption. A 30-60 mg dosage, that is just one drop, is enough to cause poisoning in an adult. It has many resourceful properties which makes it important in pharmacology. However, the fact that its consumption for the human brain is unfit remains undeniable.

The tobacco plant has been in use for centuries by various demographics for its many medicinal purposes like alleviating pain and its ability to facilitate better concentration. It is recommended in treating cognitive disorders. But recent growing addiction to it has caught the attention of health professionals, and individuals who are concerned about the many health complications it can cause. It continues to be a topic of agitated discussion and study for both, its calming and stimulating nature. However, strictly speaking considering the vulnerable present scenario, we need to be aware of the functioning and remedial strategies. Almost every other person is seen struggling to get rid of nicotine addiction. "Quit smoking" has become a popular new year's resolution and only a handful of people realise it.

But why? What is it about tobacco that you are constantly wanting to take one more puff?

Primarily, it's because in addition to the physiological impact, nicotine has a psychological impact too. It does not simply spike up your heart rate, but also influences your brain. It leads to release of endorphins from the hypothalamus located in your brain.

Wait! You must be wondering what does it all mean? Well to speak simply, endorphins are happy hormones which make you feel better and light. They are the reason why the world world becomes a better place when you light a cigarette.

Let's dive into understanding how nicotine reaches your brain and influences your mood.

Human central nervous system, which has both, parts of the brain and spinal cord, has neurotransmitters. They are the vehicles which carry messages all around the body. These passages are known as *Nicotinic Acetylcholine Receptors.* These receptors help us perform important functions like learning, development, cognitive activities, mood regulation and more. In addition to the CNS, they are found in the prefrontal cortex and hippocampus - all parts of the brain.

Nicotine combines with these receptors, opening their ion channel. Ion channels are the doors to entry and exit for outside particles inside cells. It causes a functional change in the neurotransmitters which leads to the release of sodium and calcium ions to flow into the neuron. These sudden changes lead to the release of dopamine - the reason for the immediate feeling of relief associated with reward and pleasure. Individuals want to retain the feeling of high which pushes them to keep going back to tobacco, ending up in a state of dependence and in worse cases, addiction. Once nicotine sticks to the receptors it stimulates serotonin which influences mood and immediately reduces anxiety levels. The continued use of nicotine desensitises these receptors causing mood fluctuations in the long term. And by then, the dependence is severe. As seen in therapy, such individuals show aggression, mood fluctuations, lack of concentration when deprived of nicotine.

You must know some individuals who can't function without having their daily dose of morning nicotine. People often mention that they are able to focus better, that's why they smoke at regular intervals. The reason behind this is the release of hormones like *norepinephrine* and *acetylcholine* which cause hyper attention or higher energy levels. It enables people to work longer hours with more concentration and less fatigue. The consistent use also causes synaptic plasticity, which means changes in connection between neurons. In the later chapters, we will cover these heavy terms and processes in detail.

Stable communication between neurons is crucial for healthy development of mind and body. The regular consumption of tobacco creates a trapping loop in which only nicotine feels rewarding. Other activities like socialisation, food, sports fail to compete. The trigger of hormones like endorphin and serotonin interferes with the normal mood cycles leading to more dependence and a decline on overall health. When an individual is dependent on nicotine, it disrupts their cognitive functioning and leads to problems like memory loss and poor attention due to desensitisation of the receptors. Basically, the brain becomes numb to all other feelings.

HOW DOES BRAIN-NICOTINE BONDING WORK?

Here is what happens when you consume nicotine in any form: be it cigarette, hookah or gums, it directly goes into your bloodstream. It escapes the whole intestinal passage. Meaning it does not follow the normal digestive tract. It is absorbed much faster through the bloodstream. There, it sticks to the nicotinic acetylcholine receptors which are located on the synaptic membranes of cells. We are already familiar with the process after this, which includes opening of ion channels and the release of dopamine which puts us in a strawberry state of mind. This process explains the sudden sense of pleasure one feels while smoking a cigarette or vaping . However, long and repetitive exposure to nicotine desensitises nAChRs. When consumed repeatedly people get used to it. This is the reason why, after a while, the smoke stops hitting you. People are desperately looking for ways to consume more to relish the old feeling of elevation.

The consequences of smoking are well known and highly advertised on the packages itself. One might then wonder why there have been no real attempts to curb the consumption of tobacco when its downsides are gravely numerous and pretty serious? There are many activist campaigns and health awareness programs in education and medical institutions. But they fail to make a major impact on the conscience of the smokers. Medical professionals who are well aware of the harmful effects of nicotine consumption are also trying hard to quit smoking.

Then is putting a ban on the sale of cigarettes the only solution?

Apparently as straight and clear as it looks, it is not possible. As we have learnt, tobacco has been an integral part of Indian culture which was fancied by both, the Mughals and Britishers. It is also an integral part of the economy today. ITC alone has a net income of 20751 crores. The tobacco industry has been flourshing under private industries as well as with the support of government schemes. The economy would suffer a blow in case the production is stopped or halted, generating massive unemployment. Hence, it keeps supplying you with many variants of cigarettes - mint, clove, watermelon and what not! E-cigarettes are also becoming popular. People switch to vape as an alternative, considering it is less damaging to their bodies - but at the end of the day, nicotine is nicotine, and its damage can not be undone. Since its production has become essential in generating significant revenue for the economy, we need to choose wisely as consumers for our health. You might be putting off stress at the moment but inviting long term health issues.

To highlight the issue once again, high consumption of nicotine causes a conformational change in the receptors, that means permanent, irreversible change. It desensitises them, changes the state of the ion channels, spikes up the heart rate, putting it in a state of hyper attentiveness, or gives a momentary sense of relief. As per the stats, an adolescent smokes for the first time at the age of 14-15. 90 percent of those continue to smoke till much later and become absolutely dependent on it. There are many methods of inhaling tobacco and many remedial ways for therapy. Before we start to learn about the solution, let's cover how it crosses the blood-brain barrier, leaving an imprint so strong that it ends up being an addiction. Learning about the vast impact on cognitive abilities, cellular changes, memory retention, withdrawal, and dependence will benefit our understanding of the issue. Awareness can stop addiction. Hence, continue reading ahead before you proceed for a light smoking break.

Chapter - 2
MORRIS'S MARLBORO

In 1847, in the dream city of London, Philip Morris, a teenager, opened a shop selling tobacco. It was a tiny shop on the premium Bond Street where Morris and his family tried to make an income by selling hand rolled cigarettes and loose tobacco. Their customers were elite Brits who preferred smoking luxury cigars which did justice to their well-thought superior class. The high clientele helped Philips to sustain a thriving business, giving good returns. After mastering how to roll a successful business for 8 years, Philips took the risk to start manufacturing his own cigarettes. It was indeed a daring step back in 1854 at the naive age of 21. However, it would only mark one of his many successful ventures. The tables turned in his favour. The cigarettes were a hit and soon the whole of Britain was smoking cigarettes produced by him. From 20 somethings, to people in their mid thirties, everyone was smoking Philip Morris's cigarettes. Philip created a solid legacy which was forwarded to his wife and later his brother Leopold Morris. After Philips passed away in 1873, his brother started handling the business and took it to new heights, successfully collaborating with major brands. After he took leadership of the company, Leopold registered it officially in 1885 as "**Philip Morris & Co. Ltd.**". This marked its entry in the international markets. From there, the brand was only meant to touch more heights.

With the dawn of the 20th century, the brand materialised its success in the international markets, marking a strong footprint in the United States. In 1902, the company got monumental success by launching business in the big apple city - New York. The inauguration welcomed the multitude of opportunities which helped them take charge in other markets as well. In 1954, it was launched in Australia. By this time, Philip Morris had become a giant tobacco brand, with its cigarettes being smoked around the world, the most popular and bestselling one being - Marlboro, which revolutionised the tobacco industry.

The 1900s marked the rise of Philip Morris from a small tobacco seller to the world's biggest tobacco company - Philip Morris International. Today, PMI has six multibillion brands - Dji Sam Soe launched in 1913, L&M in 1953, Longbeach in 1999, Marlboro in 1924, ST Dupont in Paris, Chesterfield in 1896 and, lastly Philip Morris which is the fourth largest international brand of the company. In the fiscal year 2023, the company was had a net income of 7813 million US dollars with 84,579 million US dollars in revenue. Throughout its lore of success, the company has faced many controversies for promoting the use of tobacco. With consistent renewal, upgradation, the company kept on improving its manufacturing process, installing the latest technology and releasing luxury products. However, the company was meant to face backlash sooner or later as its prime product was tobacco. It happened in no time, and across many countries.

SOME SHADY BUSINESS

Philip Morris repeatedly faced the blame for manipulating public health. The authorities, citizens, and activists began to highlight how the company used aggressive marketing to promote its product which had a negative impact on the health of the natives. This was seen in the United States where the company was blamed for using shady tricks to sell its products, promoting nicotine addiction. Eventually, the case was remedied by offering healthcare schemes to recover the health of the citizens. But looking at it from the larger perspective, it is pretty clear that the brand's extensive business has been damaging to the health of its consumers.

With rapid industrialization, smoking became a regular habit. It became more like a meal to be taken at fixed intervals. People smoked, not merely for a fleeting feeling of high but to kill time; during gatherings, work meetings, to add on the charisma of professionalism. The white collar employees with their luxury cigars were the standard. The habit of smoking was further glorified by Hollywood icons like James Dean, Spencer Tracy, Gary Cooper, and Audrey Hepburn. Winston Churchill was never seen without his favorite cigar. The habit was picked by the youth in an instant and by 1950s, almost 80 percent of UK was consumed in smoky air. Hence, what was first a luxury product to be used during entertainment or festivities was converted into a daily commodity - a part of the meal. It was possible to meet the high demand because of the mass production, efficient transportation, systematised warehousing, and cheap availability of resources. This sidelined the traditional way of smoking through pipes and chewing on tobacco leaves.

Philip Morris rebranded its cigarettes as the epitome of masculinity. It benefitted from gendered marketing advertising: "For man's flavour come to Marlboro Country". This raised a different market to release diverse products using tricky but smart marketing campaigns. For example, brands began producing and promoting "cigarettes for women". Smoking, thus, gained many women consumers during the 1950s. It was a culmination of marketing, launch of women-specific products, and a trend and excitement towards a "new woman"- who was modern and devoid of any social constraints.

It all seems too good to be true, making us wonder why no one is talking about the lethal consequences of smoking tobacco? Becuase back in the days there was limited awareness. However, soon people saw the emergence of articles criticising tobacco, and its viscous impact on human health. Scientists and physicians made the discovery of lung cancer and the role of cigarettes in promoting it. The growing health concerns and deaths due to tobacco raised the consciousness of the citizens. There were many campaigns to ban the sale of tobacco. The vibrant campaigning did influence people to reduce smoking making it an occasional treat, but it could not stop its sale or convince people to quit.

WHY THE "CRAZE"?

To understand the growing demand and popularity of smoking, it's important to realise its social and cultural context. As we talked about in the chapter one, all forms of consuming tobacco has held importance for the Americas. The people held it in high regard for its medical benefits, even including it in ceremonial rituals. The renowned historian Jordan Goodman, dealing with the cultural history of medicine, elaborated on the significance of tobacco for the Native americans. He talked about the "culture of dependence" and the pleasure it brings to the natives through smoking. As per studies, we have come to learn about the various medical properties of tobacco. For example, in central Mexico, it was used to treat earache. Tribes in Guatemala used it as an antiseptic and also to cure toothache. Hence, it served as both - *a tool and toxin.*

Despite the trouble of lawsuits, opposition from activists, restrictions like high tax from government, the tobacco industry is a growing industry. It has impeccable access to the market. Despite being labelled as a "toxin" product, people can't help but want one more puff. Marketing is one thing, but the real magic happens inside your brain which pushes you to consume more. You see, a human body is full of wonderful mechanics. It has in-built systems to protect itself against any kind of toxin you take. Similarly, it has a whole Blood-Brain Barrier (BBB) system to ensure that your brain gets the right nutrition and remains free of toxins like nicotine. The BBB is a semipermeable membrane of closely packed cells and tissues. It is a well connected network of blood vessels which allows the flow of nutrition and other fundamental functions. To say it simply, it is like a firewall kicking out harmful viruses/toxins. This membrane allows easy entry of oxygen, water, carbon dioxide, and other nutrients into the brain. This nature of the membrane is essential to maintain the brain's chemical balance. A perfect way to give access to good particles while kicking out the harmful substances.

But, how does it do so? How does it differentiate between "good" and "bad" particles?

Well, here we go - the membrane is made up of tightly packed endothelial cells which prevent the entrance of drugs. They basically block one entrance and push them to use a different route known as transcellular route. The scientist Paul Ehrlich conducted an experiment discovering the functioning of the Blood Brain Barrier. In this, he used a blue dye concluding that the dye spread to the rest of the body but not to the brain. Amazing, right!?

Along with the brain capillary endothelium, the BBB also has several other cells including pericytes, an astrocyte end foot, and several neural endings. This intact structure ensures that no toxin enters the brain. Many enzyme reactions happen inside this delicate membrane. They are like the floor manager of our brains making sure that every particular settles at the right place. They take help from efflux transporters to move a compound out from a cell. Consider it more like a bodyguard of the cell kicking out harmful particles. They are found in other parts of the body. Some of them are Breast Cancer Resistant Protein (BCRP), P-glycoprotein (PGP) and multiple resistance associated protein (MRP).

If these cells don't stick together, our brain can be under high risk of damage from toxins. The lack of these tight junctions allow the entry of some drugs which would have been blocked otherwise. The process through which the brain reacts to drug intake is through the *free drug hypothesis.* The discovery of this barrier has put in front a vital question of pharmacology as it restricts the entry of medicinal drugs which are necessary for the brain. In the same way, when you consume tobacco through any form, to reach the brain it needs to cross the blood brain barrier.

But like it has been said, there are exceptions, and this includes the nicotine molecule.

FREE ACCESS TO THE NICOTINE MOLECULE

The nicotine molecule is easily able to pass through the Blood-Brain Barrier. There are multiple reasons for its easy passage. The first one being its physical size. Nicotine is a tiny molecule weighing approximately 162 daltons. Its small size makes it easier for the molecule to cross through the tightly secure pack of cells. Now, if you remember, one of the properties of nicotine is high lipophilicity making it fat soluble. This makes it easier to dissolve in BBB, since BBB is rich in lipids. Also, nicotine does not rely on the transporters to travel through the bloodstream. They travel independently using passive diffusion which doesn't require significant energy. Thus it is absorbed rapidly as quick as 7-10 seconds. This is much faster than other substances.

Parts of the brain like Ventral Tegmental Area and nucleus accumbens are rich in lipids. Being fat soluble, nicotine is easily accumulated in these areas. The areas are associated with achievement and addiction, continuously stimulating the feeling of reward and dopamine. Through inhalation, the nicotine does not enter the intestinal passage. It gets directly infused into the bloodstream through the alveoli in lungs. But when you chew the leaves or gums, it travels through the mucous membrane. This is the intestinal tract, hence it dissolves comparatively slower. Its absorption is influenced by factors like pH levels, blood flow, and concentration of the nicotine.

The better the blood flow in the brain, the rapid the absorption.

Similarly the higher the amount you inhale, the better the high.

Now once it's through the BBB what happens next? Where does it go?

Easy - in your Central Nervous System. With its entry inside your brain through the barrier, it combines with the receptors - nAChRs. As we have learned, these receptors are located in the CNS and are sensitive to nicotine. Nicotine tricks these receptors changing their activity.

BRAIN LOOP

To understand it thoroughly, let's see how nicotine travels through the brain once it's inside.

Once it binds with the receptors in the *Ventral Tegmental Area,* it stimulates dopamine - the immediate feeling of pleasure you feel. This feeling of high becomes the reason for addiction. Smokers are anxious to experience the happiness induced by tobacco. Next is the activation of nAChRs in the *nucleus accumbens* region. This happens because of the release of dopamine in the VTA. It enhances the overall experience of dopamine, keeping the person hooked and wanting to go for the next puff. Next it goes to the prefrontal cortex. Here the nAChRs handle the cognitive processes. When the nicotine reaches this part, it enhances your attention span, memory, ability to focus. Hence you get a quick boost to function better and think better, enhancing your dopamine and creativity. Next it travels to *hippocampus* where it leads to changes in the synaptic plasticity - basically changing the wiring of your brain. First there is fluctuation in attention span, processing the movements, but consistent exposure may cause a damaging impact, leading to an impairment the cognitive functions.

Then it goes to *amygdala* where it influences your emotional state which also includes how you manage your stress. It can decrease the stress for the moment and make you feel elevated, but on the other hand, it can also put you in a state of nausea. Once you are dependent, and the short term dopamine is gone, it heightens stress, especially during withdrawals. *Hypothalamus* is the next stop which regulates your appetite and also your body temperature by regulating metabolic processes. After smoking, the appetite is suppressed. People who smoke frequently can not comprehend their appetite appropriately leading to sudden weight loss. *Straitum* is the last station. It handles motor control in the body. Nicotine causes a positive influence, leading to high energy and better motor performance without causing fatigue. A4b2 is the most commonly found receptor in the brain. Nicotine first activates them releasing nicotine, serotonin, norepinephrine, which affects your mood, cognitive activity, memory, motor functions and more. Then it desensitises them leading to you wanting more and more nicotine to carry on the functions. To meet the demands, more nAChRs are produced and right here, the cycle of addiction is formed. To help you understand clearly, here is a flowchart:

nACHRs → VTA → NUCLEUS ACCUMBENS → PREFRONTAL CORTEX

↓

STRAITUM ← HYPOTHALAMUS ← AMYGDALA ← HIPPOCAMPUS

Do keep in mind that these glands carry out other vital functions to keep your body and brain in sync. The process above explains how nicotine travels through the brain, impacting its various sub parts. However, in the long term, the consequences multiply, causing irreparable damage to these parts which pass down to the body as well. We can't see it immediately, but regular consumption does alter how our brain functions. It changes its cellular structure known as synaptic plasticity, and most times, it is not for the better. Marlboro might light up your mood, but it's hallowing your insides, directly attacking your nervous system.

Chapter – 3
A FERTILITY CRISIS

Every day a column, a tab, or a small headline delivers the unfortunate news of the people who died because of using tobacco. Under health columns, the side effects of smoking tobacco are featured weekly - ***"Every Cigarette You Smoke Reduces 22 Minutes of Your Life: Reveals Research"***. There are dozens of interviews available on youtube of smokers who regret touching cigarettes as they count their final days wearing an oxygen mask, crumpled in a hospital bed, dying of cancer or other fatal condition caused by tobacco. The numbers are everywhere, urgently conveying a warning to us to take reasonable actions. The sheer number of diagnoses and deaths do not seem enough to convince people to quit smoking. 62.9 million people above the age of 15 smoke tobacco products in the USA alone, making it the fourth top country when it comes to smoking. Although the trends show a decline in consumers because of more awareness, the population engaged in consuming tobacco remains exposed to the consequences.

Nicotine is notorious for causing innumerable health related problems. Respiratory issues, multiple cancers, mental fog are the well known issues but there are many other health irregularities caused by nicotine which can disrupt your daily life. As we have already seen, it is a toxin known for its ability to interfere with the blood brain barrier - the firewall of brain. On top of it, it has also proven to be carcinogenic, often leading to cancer diagnosis in the long term. This is the reason that even though the declining number of smokers seems like a relief, it's not the end of the problem. Out of the huge number mentioned above, almost 16 million smokers end up getting diagnosed with COPD, a respiratory illness which has no definite cure. **Chronic Obstructive Pulmonary Disease** or COPD damages the lungs by directly impacting the airways. The obstruction in the airway passage makes it difficult to breathe comfortably. The initial symptoms look completely harmless like coughing, mucus, wheezing, or shortness of breath. Over some time, the person feels an overall decline in health like muscle loss, chest pressure, weight loss, restlessness, infections and more. That's when their conscience hits that it's not just a regular cough and there is a rush for a doctor's appointment. The number stated above might be an underestimation since most people are not even aware of it.

A FATAL COUGH

COPD is a fatal disease and one of its leading causes is smoking tobacco. So let's break down the enigma of this fatal respiratory disease.

COPD is the culmination of progressive lung diseases, which slowly and quietly destroys the air sacs of your lungs.

Result?

Interference with your blood flow causing disruption in distribution of particles. Meaning, it allows more particulars to gather in the sacs like water. It also inclues chronic bronchitis meaning inflammation. This directly causes obstruction in oxygen passage. With obstructions and less space in the tube passage, the mucus is jammed. You must know the irritating feeling of a blocked nose. The mucus does not allow the air to pass, leading to laboured breath, runny nose, and exhaustion. At this stage, it looks like a regular cold - harmless, curable, temporary. However, when the condition is left untreated for considerable time, its progression follows. By the time most people fix a check up, the illness has towered, causing huge damage to your insides. It can cause many critical infections and heart problems. The effect is not just physiological. With worsening of the disease, you might feel mental confusion, stagnation, and even brain fog. After all, it is hard to think and talk clearly when you have to cough every minute. Thus, it can become hard for a person to focus, perform daily activities without feeling fatigue, keep track of activities and so on.

This condition is also influenced by age. After the age of 40, if an individual is engaged in chain smoking accompanied by a poor lifestyle, the chances of developing COPD increases significantly. In case you have other health issues like asthma or diabetes the risk is even greater. Living in an environment polluted with chemicals, fumes, mold, toxins, poorly ventilated homes, access to no clean air, can also cause COPD. This benign disease is the 4th leading factor of deaths globally. Funny how COVID got all our attention, whereas COPD has been silently killing people for years.

WOMEN, WOMBS, AND NICOTINE

When it comes to smoking tobacco, the list of consequences is long. Smoking gives rise to many related diseases - from cancer being the most common one to heart diseases, diabetes, vision loss, reproductive health issues, problems with the immune system, gum diseases like periodontitis, aortic aneurysm and more. Its impact on women's reproductive health has also attracted wide concern. Given that young women are picking up cigarettes more, it's important to spread awareness about the long term health consequences they might face.

Tobacco consumption has proved to have a detrimental impact, reducing the fertility rate in women, making it hard to conceive as well as leading to many other hormonal changes. The side effects of smoking cigarettes are not gendered. Men are equally in danger as hyper consumption of smoking can harm the DNA of the sperm.

The alarming effects of smoking puts pregnant women under more danger. It is strictly advised to avoid tobacco and alcohol during pregnancy. Tobacco is not only harmful for the mother, but its toxins can also influence the unborn baby. Despite the health awareness and advice from doctors, the number of mothers who are in contact with tobacco smoke surprises us. Almost **400,000** infants come in contact with smoking even before they are born. These numbers represent only one country - the US. The data gets worse for developing countries.

In countries like India, pregnant women who work on fields are usually found in more critical condition. Their daily life in poverty fueled regions involve hard physical labour, spending long hours in front of woodfire smoke, or chemically polluted air. The smoke from the *bidi* is damaging to the health of pregnant women. The lack of resources and medical help, makes the delivery harder, leaving the lives of mother and newborn in danger. Hence, be it the mother smoking nicotine, or the secondhand smoke, any sort of tobacco contact is damaging to the health of the newborn. It interferes with fetal development, sometimes leading to stillbirth. Women are also prone to cervical cancer and the cases are concerningly high. Pregnancy, menstruation, lactation, and menopause makes women more vulnerable to the harsh impacts of smoking.

Women's health is consistently at a risk as their monthly cycle bears the brunt. Studies have shown that women who actively smoke are likely to experience dysmenorrhoea. It is a condition of painful menstruation accompanied by heavy bleeding. The hormonal imbalances can also lead to early menopause, causing an upheaval in hormones and physical health. The shift becomes harder to adapt with night sweats and hot flashes. Young women experience irregular/reduced periods, or reduced duration of the flow which means a shorter follicular phase.

It might surprise you that a mother's smoking habit influences the menstruation cycle of the daughter! Studies have shown girls getting an early menarche, or the onset of periods, when exposed to smoke in the womb. A study by The American Society for Reproductive Medicine has shown that about 13 percent of women become infertile because of heavy smoking. Male gametes also experience damage because of frequent smoking. Studies have backed up the claim that smoking causes a decrease in semen volume and quality. Dozens of reports are available on the internet, on websites talking about the damage in DNA or chromosomal changes caused by consuming tobacco. In the long term, if you are thinking of starting a family, it is important to take into account your health and overall lifestyle. Creating a smoke and nicotine free environment will only contribute to your overall well being.

Women planning to give birth need to be conscious of their consumption of tobacco in the long term. A preparatory period is required by your body, otherwise the risk of miscarriages and stillbirth are high. It has been proven in multiple studies that female smokers have a low number of oocytes, shortening the reproductive cycle. With low oocytes, that is the female gamete, the chances of it maturing into a fertile egg are less too. Advanced medical technology has increased the chances of becoming parents through many other methods in which the to-be mother doesn't have to undergo the period of gestation, delivery, and labour. There is the option for surrogacy where the surrogate carries the child for the intended parents. IVF is a popular option with every other couple considering it a safe way of having babies. In this process, the fertilisation of the egg and sperm happens in a medical laboratory and then is inserted inside the uterus of the intended mother. The babies born through this process are popularly known as lab babies. It leads to efficient conception but does not ensure a successful gestation period or delivery. In assisted pregnancies as well, it is vital to ensure there is no consumption of tobacco. Thus, absolute reliance on only medical technology is risky. It's best to avoid being ignorant and listen to our bodies.

Teenagers today are more sexually active compared to the last decades. To practice safe sex, people rely on contraceptives. Some of the popular ways of avoiding an unwanted pregnancy are wearing a condom and being on birth control. In case of condom failures, many people opt for the quick fix - oral contraceptive, also known as "morning pill". The oral birth pill control consists of the hormone oestrogen which prevents pregnancy. Oral birth control is infamous for causing hormonal imbalances, which causes issues with conceiving later. It causes a multitude of other problems like inflammation, hair loss, stress, mental anxiety, bad gut health and more. Out of these side effects, one of the most serious ones is the risk of ovarian cancer and infertility. If a woman takes ipill and tobacco both regularly, it puts her at a 20 times higher risk of developing coronary heart diseases. The risk of a stroke and haemorrhage is also higher. The data presented by the 2014 US Surgeon General report says ED and vasospasm is a recurring complaint in men. There are reports that have claimed that nicotine hinders required blood flow in the genitals but there is no credible data to back it up.

This, women need to be aware of any changes in their menstrual cycle, especially if they engage in regular smoking. You see, a woman's menstrual cycle is sensitive to abrupt changes like sudden exhaustion, hormonal imbalances, prolonged periods of trauma, lifestyle changes and more. For a healthy cycle, it is crucial to look after your habits, avoid consumption of foods which can alter the cycle, and avoid consumption of alcohol and tobacco. When ultra processed foods can have a damaging effect, then nicotine, which is an identified carcinogenic toxin, can have a lethal impact on your reproductive health. It is important to understand how nicotine interferes with your monthly cycle and alters its flow, duration and other relevant hormones.

NICOTINE THROUGHOUT THE 28-DAY CYCLE

The female menstrual cycle in humans has four phases: menstrual (1-5 days), follicular phase (1-13 days), ovulation phase (14-21 days), and luteal phase (22-28 days). Let's study each phase of this cycle and how nicotine affects it.

The first phase lasts for about a week during which the uterine lining sheds. It is characterised by high progesterone and estrogen levels. Smoking during this phase interrupts the blood flow. The uterus tries its best to keep the balance and ensure adequate blood flow. This increases the prostaglandin levels, causing severity of cramps, making them more painful than regular periods. In alternative cases, it enhances the blood flow, causing heavier periods than usual known as menorrhagia. The bottom line is that nicotine activity and women hormones don't get along very well.

The next phase is about two weeks long, overlapping with the last of the menstruation period. During this phase, the oocyte, the female gamete, matures into ovum for fertilisation. Follicle stimulating hormone manages the maturing of the egg. This period is also marked by high estrogen levels. Smoking has a detrimental impact on the eggs, reducing both the quality and number of eggs. Nicotine disrupts the production of estrogen causing an imbalance which delays the development of follicles causing a delay in the menstrual cycle.

Next, ovulation happens when the mature egg is released. This period is accompanied by a surge in the luteinizing hormone. Smoking tobacco confuses the hormonal signals for the release of the egg which can cause irregular cycles. Tobacco also causes oxidative stress which can impair the eggs.

The next and the final stage of the cycle is the luteal phase. It is characterised by high levels of progesterone which again brick the uterus lining. The uterus does this to prepare for any potential pregnancy. Smoking brings a drop in the progesterone level causing shortening of the phase. This has a direct impact on the potential implantation. It triggers worse premenstrual syndrome also known as PMS. It is accompanied by mood swings, fatigue, bloating and imbalances in hormones like serotonin which is responsible for balancing the mood. Hence for a regulated, well balanced, mind-body synced lifestyle, it is important to regulate nicotine consumption. Otherwise as mentioned above, it can pave way to many unthought imbalances which can cause long term health consequences. Enhanced treatments are available as an option, but the ancient saying sticks - prevention is better than cure.

MEN, FERTILITY AND DAMAGE

The consumption of tobacco is equally detrimental to the reproductive health of men. For men, it puts them at a high risk of erectile dysfunction and prostate cancer. This happens because of a simple mechanism. Taking nicotine in any form narrows blood vessels throughout the body, including the penis. With restricted blood supply, it becomes hard for the penis to be in the state of erection ending up in ED. Nicotine is also a vasoconstrictor that constricts the blood vessels disrupting the supply of blood throughout the organs. It also decreases the nitric oxide which causes vasodilation, that is widening of blood vessels.

Vasodilation maintains the engorgement of penis. It can cause both arteriogenic ED caused by constriction of vessels and neurogenic ED caused by irregularities in nerves related to pleasure. An article published in the journal *Andrologia* confirmed that smoking can triple the chances of ED. This data was confirmed in another study by the *American Journal of Preventive Medicine* in 2022. It mentions that consuming nicotine in between 20-65 ages increases the chances of ED. It is also dose dependent, however, every puff is causing damage to your body somewhere.

Consumption of tobacco can pave way for a painful health journey whose downsides you start seeing once you cross the fit age of 30. It opens doors for many unwanted conditions which can chip at your finances and also cause huge damage to your health, mental stress, and in worse cases death. COPD, struggle with conceiving, infertility, irregular periods, ED, cancers are some of the long term side effects which smokers grapple with. As discussed in the earlier chapters, its toxins start affecting the human mind the second we consume tobacco, leading to a change in the mental state. With regular inhalation, your body also begins to show the downsides. Most times, the damage done can not be undone. Thus, catch a breath, think twice, *who's consuming whom?*

Chapter – 4
BRAIN GAME, OR BLAME DAMAGE?

The legend of the Marlboro Man is recalled vividly, but where is this epitome of masculinity today? Apparently, the last time it was seen was in 1999 and since then it is grieving a legal defeat, after struggling, suffering, and losing to lawsuits. It was a product of the giant tobacco company, Philip Morris, which was blamed for running a highly profitable business at the cost of its consumers' health. Its most popular ad campaign, "Marlboro Man", took it to towering popularity, but also brought to attention the wicked strategies, false claims, misleading information, all of which the company was using to attract more consumers to smoke tobacco. The ads targeted a global consumer group, despite their age and health background, not taking into account the critical illnesses they may have had. By directly attracting the consciousness of the young consumers, the brand was found guilty of using aggressive marketing for producing and promoting a toxin which was toying with the citizens' health. Philip Morris had to deal with the consequences which came with defamation, downs in business and heavy compensation to the victims…but not defeat.

PROFITS VS PUBLIC HEALTH

Some of the cases which brought the world's watchful gaze were the **Florida Cases** where four US states - Florida,

Minnesota, Mississippi, and Texas reached a settlement with the tobacco companies. It manifested in the form of a compensation and them obliging to follow responsible manufacturing and business practices. However, the case which is lauded for shaking the tobacco industry is the **Master Settlement Agreement.** The case goes back to 1998 where major tobacco companies finally faced the ugly truth of their negligible practices. MSA is the largest civil litigation settlement in US history. The agreement was between the companies and 46 states, the District of Columbia, and five US territories. The companies against which the cases were filed are some of the most renowned names - Philip Morris, RJ Reynolds, Brown & Williamson, and Lorillard. In addition to these companies, other associations that got their hands dirty in supporting the trade of tobacco were also involved in the legal hearings.

The case proved revolutionary in the tobacco industry in the US. It ended up fining billions of dollars as compensation from these big companies for the damage caused by loss of life. The deaths caused due to smoking had a negative impact on the local economy for which the state asked for remuneration. Part of the total sum went into creating an independent awareness organisation to educate the youth about the consequences of tobacco, promote anti-smoking campaigns, and help people to overcome their decades old addiction. The agreement asked for stricter procedures for the production, branding and advertising of cigarettes. The state also implemented an age restriction. The companies were prohibited to sell tobacco to minors - individuals below 18 years of age. Cartoons in cigarette advertising were banned to stop any misleading information. Attempts were made to reduce the visibility of the product in the market.

Advertising through huge billboards and public transit were strictly prohibited. The trade of tobacco was separated from other merchandise so that the public remained conscious of the consequences.

The agreement was led by the American states. Citizens were active observants. The money received from the companies went into treating smoking related illnesses and maintaining the health of citizens. It was a happy end where the taxpayers got prolonged justice for their health. The agreement was finalised in November, 1998. Since then many other tobacco companies have also joined the agreement to practice ethical business, but deep down secretly hoping to avoid scary lawsuits. The exposure of many important documents which highlighted how the companies had been hiding important research related to nicotine use changed the attitude of the natives. The consumers were overwhelmed by mistrust resulting in reduced sales of cigarettes. Alas, if only lawsuits could stop the addiction!

There are several other cases where the victims took the courage to sue the companies for selling carcinogenic toxins like nicotine under false advertising. One such case which went viral was the **Cipollone Case** in the 1980s. The plaintiff, Rose Cipollene, suffered a painful death due to lung cancer which she developed from smoking tobacco. The young Rose started smoking when she was merely 16, which took her life at 58. Her husband sued the cigarette brand which her wife smoked after she passed away. It might look like an emotional, irrational step, but let me tell you, it was not in vain. His courageous lawsuit led to justice for his late wife. In 1988, the jury in New Jersey awarded an impressive sum of 400,000 dollars to the husband for his loss. The verdict was based on the reason that till 1966, the company did not in fact warn its consumers that the product is harmful for health and can cause deadly diseases like cancer. The company also also claimed that smoking its cigarettes, which were made of tobacco, was "safe". A hysterical irony!

It was a monumental yet short lived victory as the case verdict was reversed in 1992. However, till this date, the case holds immense significance. Thousands of people have lost their lives to tobacco. Cases like these force us to introspect and inspect the blunders of the companies and figure out, if as consumers, we are being exploited. The company's internal documents were exposed in which it deliberately hid the side effects of consuming its products. There have been many other instances which revealed that since the beginning, these businesses were aware of the addictive nature of nicotine but kept the public in dark and profited at the cost their health. Smoky business, indeed!

GLOBAL WAVE

This wave which started from the USA spread globally where the concern of the citizens exposed the malpractices of tobacco manufactures in their own countries. Many battles were won, but there were unfortunate defeats as well. Margaret McTear sued Imperial Tobacco for the death of her husband due to lung cancer, but she lost the case. In Canada, major companies like Imperial Tobacco, JTI-Macdonald, and Rothmas had to pay 15 billion dollars as compensation. In Australia as well, the government made strict packaging mandatory with clear labels. Every concerning voice helped move a file bringing home justice to families who lost their dear ones.

These cases were 50 years back, when the digital media did not exist and people really did not have many means to go and learn about a product. Hence, it was important for the companies to advertise their products correctly, informing the citizens about the potential damages. The relationship between businesses and consumers was entirely based on trust. Now, in 2025, with so much information available on the internet, accessible within seconds, it is easier to learn both - how to quit and start smoking.

There are many international organisations on a drive to reduce the rate of smoking, especially among youth. Among these, the Truth Initiative is worth a check. It an institution which has been relentlessly working to educate and make the youth aware about the side effects of tobacco on health. They believe that every campaign helps save a life. It has evolved with time to make itself accessible to the digital gen-z and help them quit nicotine. It uses clinical research, sessions with medical experts, scientific methods, and credible data to craft programs where you can manage your addiction without necessarily undergoing a painful quitting journey. Awareness plays a central role in preventing the coming of age youngsters to get stuck in the loop of puffs. We know smoking kills and has killed hundreds worldwide. Its physiological side effects are often talked about. The research in the sphere has led to development of treatments which can prove to be costly but gives a second chance at life. But, the treatment can only cure the affected organs. Nicotine is known for travelling through the brain, causing upheavals in your hormones, productivity, experiences, and feelings. But, the issue is, the dopamine hit is momentary but its consequences are not.

A MIND TRICK

Recall the last chapters, where we read elaborately about how consumption of tobacco destroys the health of the smokers. Many develop lung cancer which then can spread to the throat, mouth, gums - everywhere. Fear of diseases lingers as an active threat. On top of it, it causes imbalance with hormones which can disrupt the menstrual cycle for women leading to issues in pregnancy. For men too, it paves way towards erectile dysfunction and prostate cancers. The numbers mentioned have caught the attention of the people who are actively in the fight to quit tobacco. The diseases caused are enough to make us aware of the concerning impacts. But on top of it, it leads to neurodegenerative diseases which can hit the person at any age, and there is really no cure for them. These are genetic and there is a high chance that your children might inherit them. Hence, it's not only you who suffers, but your coming generations might end up becoming innocent victim of nicotine.

So, how does this work?

Do you remember from the early chapters how nicotine travels inside your system? How it sneaks directly into the brain, wrecking the hormones on its way? From your temperament to temperature, it alters the state of your mind and body. It first takes you on a high, giving a sweet and liberating feeling. However, a devil in disguise, its long term usage wrecks your brain functioning. When the process is repeated frequently, the receptors are desensitised.

RESULT?

The ability to experience joy, the ability to focus, and think is altered. In other words, there is a high dependence on nicotine, without which it's hard to perform regular tasks. The smoker can only feel "in control" of himself, or capable of getting to work, as long as they have access to nicotine.

The reason behind is synaptic plasticity. Now we have been reading this word since start. Simply speaking, it is a change in how your brain communicates. Keep in mind, every single experience you have, things you learn, words you read, the way you interpret events have an impact on your brain. The happy, joyful, passionate activities and the stressful grim days collectively shape your brain's neural circuit. A change in brain plasticity changes the arrangement of this neural circuit. That means external activities directly affect how you process events. If you have a bad pool experience, you might feel scared to dive in next time. It is because your brain registers fear and anxiety from the event and goes on alert mode. Similarly, when you smoke, if feels happy, asking to repeat the activity.

So, how does it look inside the brain?

Technically speaking, synapse refers to the passage through which one neuron passes electrical or chemical signals to the next neuron in connection. In response to the neural activity, these synapses are modified over time. When an activity is repeatedly, and regularly performed, like learning a language, or solving quizzes, riding a bicycle, the neurons adapt to it and respond in a way to assist you when you perform that activity. You must have heard the phrase – "*train your brain*". It happens through this mechanism.

When an activity is repeatedly performed, those particular synapses become stronger, known as **long term potentiation,** and when there is a halt in the activity, they weaken, known as **long term depression**. This is primarily done to clear your brain, adapt to the new information, help you retain for the important tasks, leading to growth in a particular area. There is a popular theory that as infants, we are born with a fixed number of brain cells and carry them throughout our lives. The theory remains conflicted, many scientists agree, others have differing opinions. What stays true is that the neurons are modified as per our circumstances. The neural connections are built up over time as we meet and greet people, go through various emotions, and different experiences which alter our thinking and critical abilities. This discovery amused Santiago Ramon y Cajal - a Spanish neuroanatomist. He was the first to propose that memories are dependent on the neural connections. This interference in the neural connections also influences your memory retention. The reason for experiencing memory fog, or memory loss therefore is changes in connections. Nicotine speeds up this process, causing neurodegenerative diseases.

HELPING HANDS

The pleasure of puff is short lived, but its side effect not so short and sweet. The lawsuits above speak for the diagnosed side effects of smoking. There are other unseen, undiscovered stories where the victim feels troubled in the head, not in the body. These issues are often sidelined since the effects are not visible in the early stages. Once the synapses are damaged, that is once your brain cells or neurons stop communicating with each other effectively, hardly any treatment can bring them back to as they were. Individuals can then consult the best professionals to help manage the symptoms, but the chances of complete recovery is almost nil. The synapses are essential in maintaining all your activities, from your motor responses, to memory, to sensory functions. A disbalance in the chemical interaction leads to further serious consequences like depressive episodes, schizophrenia, Alzheimer's, Huntington's, and early aging.

For a smoker, all these issues linger at the back of the head. But like they say - better late than never. The digitally driven globalised village is full of a multitude of resources and options. If a person is trying to quit, they can be part of a community, share their journey, inspire others who are struggling, and make a better change not just for themselves, but at a society level as well. There is the option of taking help virtually from medical professionals. This way you can get the needed help even in remote areas. Individuals can be part of the hard working anti-nicotine campaigns which are trying to save the health of the youngsters.

Quitting is not a race to win. Rather, it's a more collaborative and inclusive effort. Also, remember, communication is the key for a healthy relationship. The same applies to the human body. With effective communication between the neurons, the mind and body share a long term, healthy, and thriving relationship.

Chapter – 5
PURSUIT OF HAPPINESS

"Dopamine is not about the pursuit of happiness, it is about the happiness of pursuit",

Dr. Robert Sapolsky, Neuroendocrinologist.

I would like to introduce to our readers some special people before we begin with our next discussion over tobacco and nicotine. Meet Brandon who started smoking in his mid teens and by the sweet age of 18, he was diagnosed with Buerger's disease - a rare medical condition in which the blood supply to hands and feet is blocked. Tobacco has been identified as a reason which causes this disorder. Patients can take active steps to manage the symptoms, but there is no complete recovery. As for Brandon, after 9 painful years of struggle, he ended up amputating both his legs and several fingertips. His present days are a mix of recovery and regret. Now, meet Christine - a 49-year-old woman residing in Pennsylvania, USA. She started smoking at 16 and never looked back. At 44, she was diagnosed with oral cancer, leading to the removal of her lower jaw. She is doing better, but what's lost is lost.

Such examples can be found everywhere. The cases are numerous. You don't have to google these stories, they live and breathe in our neighbourhood, in our families. But we fail to bring about any change, apart from some momentary pity towards the victim. The stories stay in our consciousness for a moment, but the next minute, we are gripped by the same cycle - back to square one. The belief is that we can escape the matrix, that the poison of nicotine won't affect *us* so brutally. The tricky question is: How do we get stuck in this loop of cigarette smoking? What happens after that first puff that going back seems like such a tempting idea? The first smoke is often a result of pressure from friends, as a way of engaging in fun, in an attempt to fuel young adrenaline, to embrace masculinity and freedom, and so on. Most of these people, however, stick to the habit eternally. Some pick it up to cope with stress whereas others try to keep chasing the high which is triggered by the increased levels dopamine. In the end, our hormones become dependent on nicotine, signalling the brain to "get more."

A HORMONAL HAVOC

The term "hormones" tends to give us a jump scare. In our daily life, we encounter plenty of irregularities caused due to hormonal imbalance - acne marks, pimples, inflammation, mood swings, severe diseases like thyroid, fluctuations in menstrual cycle and the list continues. It is, thus, essential for the hormones to be in sync, function well, and get exposed to a suitable environment in order to avoid the above issues and have balanced and regulated days. Another fun fact: Human body have *over 50 hormones*. A hormone is available for every situation - cortisol for stress, adrenaline for emergencies, dopamine and serotonin for happiness and joy, insulin for maintaining glucose levels, TSH for thyroid, progesterone and oestrogen for maintaining a healthy menstrual cycle, etc. Once the normal biological hormonal regulation is disturbed, it takes a lengthy, troublesome, expensive process to bring them back on track. Hormonal acne, PCOS, diabetes are a few examples which come with lifetime liability of treatment, but no definite cure. The best option which then remains is to keep the situation under control. However, regulating the hormones in itself is tricky, involving endless rounds to the doctor, never ending medicines, and a strain on your pocket.

The disturbances to hormones can be due to external, internal, or genetic factors. With genes involved, the risk of disorders is relatively higher and not entirely in our hands to stop. External factors give more hope. There, we can actively participate in creating a lifestyle in which the external environment does not trigger or disturb our hormone levels. Some of the standards to maintain a healthy, balanced lifestyle would be, as the norm says - eat homemade food, move regularly, walk to support your heart, meditation for the mind, remove processed foods, reduce alcohol, and without a second thought - **Quit Smoking**. There is no rule of exception when it comes to smoking tobacco, and smoking alone is responsible for causing a multitude of issues ranging from minor interruptions in your mood to fatal diseases.

UNDERSTANDING DOPAMINE DUALITY

Nicotine has been identified as the cause behind numerous imbalances in the hormones in the Central Nervous System. One of the hormones which is severely affected is dopamine. Dopamine, popularly known as the "happy hormone", has dual functionality. It is both a hormone and a neurotransmitter and it does so much more than just influencing our moods. We will be covering in detail its relevance and the possible disorders its imbalance can cause.

Dopamine is a fascinating molecule in the human brain. It acts as a chemical messenger, regulating our moods, motivation, reward feeling, validation, pleasure and more.

During regular check ups, we often sideline it, undermining its significance. However, fluctuations in its levels can take a toll on our mental health. The lifestyle today is surrounded by exposure to high levels of stress, an environment full of toxins, foods laden with chemicals, and an unhealthy amount of screen time.

These activities disrupt the chemical balance and neural circuits, limiting the range of experiencing life. Dopamine influences a diverse range of mechanisms in our body beyond the simple feeling of experiencing joy. First is its well known function associated with the reward system in our brains. It is stimulated by performing activities which interest us or participating in some standard fun activities like going for movies, playing sports, eating one's favourite foods etc. To experience that particular feeling, individuals keep on recreating similar events and activities to feel more pleasure. This simple mechanism excites our curiosity.

Do we really need this hormone to carry out a regular, balanced life? After all, not being able to eat your favorite foods should not be fatal, right? Well, not immediately, but over time, everything leaves a mark.

Dopamine has a role in helping humans carry out their basic behaviours which includes eating and reproducing. It also plays an active role in maintaining coordinated physical movement. It stays in contact with *basal ganglia* - a small part located deep inside the brain. It coordinates with the brain and together, they carry on voluntary movements like picking a pen, throwing a ball, etc. In absence of adequate or imbalanced dopamine, individuals are exposed to many possible movement disorders, including Parkinson's disease. Parkinson also falls into the category of diseases with no chance of recovery. It is characterised by tremors, stiffness and difficulty in executing movements.

The reason behind it?

Degeneration of dopamine producing neurons in a key area of the brain - *substantia nigra* which is located in the midbrain.

Another function dopamine performs is maintaining ambition and motivation. Hence during periods of low dopamine, it's hard to get out of bed, to focus, and execute tasks throughout the day. It leads to pent up frustration, discomfort, and irritation. Digital media offers cheap ways to experience a dopamine rush through engaging in scrolling, binge watching movies, etc. In a short time, these sources of entertainment become more taxing than relaxing. The trending terms used to describe these behaviours are *"bedrotting"* or *"doom scrolling"*. They reflect how social media has disbalanced our dopamine levels.

But how are smoking and doom scrolling related? They complement each other, worsening dopamine levels. As a result, individuals are victims of two addictions: Nicotine and doom scrolling. Both of these cause short term dopamine boost making our brain lag later. Where its insufficiency can lead to lack of motivation and many mental disorders like depression, its excess is no good either. Unregulated high dopamine levels can end up in conditions like schizophrenia or hallucinations.

WHEN THE BALANCE TIPS...

Apart from the motor movements, dopamine also plays a role in strengthening your memory. It tells your brain what you like. It builds the neural circuit as per your desires. This is how the human brain makes decisions - analysing the satisfaction level of the end result. Besides these, we need it throughout our lives - to show excitement of having an ice cream, the happiness of seeing an old friend, or on receiving a good grade. It pushes us to find out more and explore our interests in pursuit of the euphoric feeling. Its significance can not be understated when it comes to keeping the brain chemicals in harmony. An imbalance can trigger multiple disorders for most of which, science has not been able to find a treatment. To name a few, we have Obsessive Compulsive Disorder, Depression, Dopamine Dysregulation Syndrome, Tourette Syndrome, Restless Leg Syndrome, Attention Deficit Hyperactivity Disorder, etc. All these happen because dopamine's job is not only to make you happy, it is also a neurotransmitter and hence ensures correct signalining, transfer of information and movement. Maybe that is why the saying goes: "Laughter is the best medicine". Because a crises in dopamine can give you a lot of trouble.

AN ANAMOLY

Let's rewind back a little. Do you remember nicotinic acetylcholine receptors from chapter 1? Let's summarise it briefly. nAChRs is a subset of receptors in the brain. They respond to the neurotransmitter, acetylcholine. These receptors are present in the Central Nervous System including the Ventral Tegmental Area which is associated with reward processing. It regulates your stress, learning, memory retention, signalling for motor movements and also addiction. The nicotine molecule easily crosses the blood brain barrier and binds with the nAChRs receptors, travelling through the whole brain including the VTA. These regions are laden with dopamine producing neurons known as *dopaminergic neurons.* While passing by, nicotine stimulates these neurons to produce dopamine. The dopamine produced is released in the Nucleus Accumbens which handles the feelings of joy, pleasure, and happiness. With continued exposure, the receptors become used to the experience of happiness caused by nicotine intake. It also desensitises the receptors leading to an unhealthy reliance. Hence, for the smoker, to experience the emotions of liberation and joy, more nicotine consumption becomes a priority.

This experience is further amplified by the inhibition of *GABAergic* neurons. As the name suggests, these neurons produce gamma-aminobutyric acid (GABA). Their main fucntion is to limit the dopamine release in the brain. When suppressed, they can not stop the release. As result, the chemical balance is disturbed and it confuses the brain and interferes with decision making.

To explain this in a more simplified way, nicotine hijacks your brain's reward pathway. It creates a momentary mirage of euphoria, luring the smoker to keep on taking more puffs. This continued reliance on nicotine consumption to "feel better" or "think clearly" ends up being an addiction which often comes with high cravings to inhale more. It brings immediate satisfaction and gratification. One does not need to be an addict to experience the withdrawal symptoms. If you are a regular smoker, you must have experienced a drop in your energy levels and low mood phases with a drop in nicotine levels. It becomes hard to realise the same level of happiness through any other activity like socialisation, sports, or foods, since the reward pathway is dependent on nicotine.

MAPPING THE 4 PATHWAYS

Let's take a look at how nicotine disrupts the reward pathways of the brain. There is not just one fixed route when it comes to happiness. There are four dopaminergic pathways which ensure smooth and sufficient regulation of dopamine which further govern functions like mood regulation, motor movements, feelings of appreciation, validation and more.

First is the ***nigrostriatal pathway***: It is a dopamine dependent route which maintains voluntary movement and balance. Its origin is in the midbrain stretching upto the striatum. This route starts and stops motor movement. Parkinsons disease is one side effect of damage in this pathway.

The second, ***tuberoinfundibular pathway*** connects the hypothalamus to the pituitary gland. In this route, dopamine is released in the hypothalamus. The dopamine is essential for the inhibition of prolactin in the pituitary gland. Prolactin is essential in the development of breasts and milk production. This pathway regulates physiological functions like cognitive movements, learning and more. The dopamine route is affected by medicinal drugs which can disrupt the receptors, leading to blockage of dopamine and a sudden increase in prolactin. High prolactin hormone leads to breast enlargement, galactorrhea, and sexual dysfunction.

The third pathway, ***mesocortical pathway,*** is also located inside the brain and connects the ventral tegmental area to the prefrontal cortex. It handles primary functions like attention, concentration, verbal memory, arousal, constructing emotional response and more. The pathway is sensitive to the drug intake because of a trigger in the dopamine. An imbalance or irregularities in the route causes disorders like schizophrenia.

The last is the ***mesolimbic pathway*** which is associated with the feeling of reward, appreciation, and pleasure. This route is highly dopamine dependent which signals for the rewarding behaviours. Understanding this route is most important, as it is significantly influenced by the consumption of toxins like nicotine. The route runs between the ventral tegmental area located in the midbrain to the nucleus accumbens in the basal forebrain. VTA is the starting point of the route which signals the activation of the reward mechanism. The dopamine produced targets the nucleus accumbens which translates the signals into the feeling of pleasure and motivation. It also influences other regions like amygdala which carries emotional aspects of rewards, prefrontal cortex which analyzes the value of the reward and helps to take a decision on it.

The last is ***hippocampus*** which stores memories of your experiences. An anomaly in this pathway leads to substance use disorders which leads to high dependence on nicotine. During periods of withdrawals, enough dopamine is not produced which can lead to *anhedonia,* meaning inability to feel joy. In some cases it can develop into depression. In case the dopamine levels shoot up, it ends up in hallucinations or schizophrenia - another mental disorder with little to no chances of recovery.

HINT TOWARDS HOPE

Research centres, government bodies and NGOs, have conducted many field studies, interviewing people, studying behaviours on how nicotine has affected the regular smokers. *The National Health and Nutrition Examination Survey* examined the link between smoking and depression. The study was conducted between 1999-2004. The researchers studied both smokers and non-smokers and their association with mental problems like depression and anxiety. The report concluded that females who smoked suffered from depression more than the females who do not engage in smoking. They also showed higher symptoms of panic disorders, high possibility of severe impairment and more. Male smokers showed a narrow difference in depression and anxiety in comparison to non smokers. Concerning data confronts us that shows children start smoking as early as middle school, before puberty. **5.2 percent** of middle school students smoke as and when they can arrange. **17.2 percent** of high schoolers are regular smokers. **90 percent** of smokers take their first try before turning 20. Now we know the "how" of nicotine's effect on our bodies.

The chapter is a humble reminder to cut down on digital and toxic shortcuts which are constantly triggering chemical imbalance in your brains. The above passages have shown in detail how nicotine can lead to incurable diseases and it's just the tip of the iceberg. One can google to find the endless number of families who have lost someone to tobacco. Those who survived paid a price, and life truly was never the same for them. The stories are of survival, reminding all of us to make healthy choices for ourselves.

Chapter - 6
NICORETTE

We have one big question looming in front of us: **"How do I quit!?"**

We know now, where nicotine comes from, how we use it, and the overall impact it has on our lives. We are aware of its addictive nature. But is there a solution? How can we break the loop of the cycle of cigarettes? What are the right ways and how much do they work? Well, catch your breath, it's time to look at the solution.

Everyday we meet people who try again and again to quit, but often give up. It is very important to take small hopeful steps towards quitting. They make small lifestyle changes, like grabbing a snack after lunch instead of a smoke. Quitting nicotine might seem like a mountain at first. However, today we have access to many alternative products which can make it a bearable experience. *Nicotine Replacement Therapy* is one such feasible and accessible solution. It has proven to reduce cravings with a success rate of 55 percent. Impressive, right? It is a go to go option for many people. Most of the NRT products can be bought over the counter.

So, what is Nicotine Replacement Therapy and how reliable and effective is it? Who has access to it? How much, when and for how long?

NRT products were first seen in the market in the 1970s. A Swedish company, Leo AB, launched *Nicorette* gums. It was the first NRT product - an effort by Ove Fernö, earning him the title of the founding father of modern pharmacotherapy for smoking. The gums were loved by people. They started consuming them as an alternative option, given the less amount of nicotine in them. In a decade, NRTs were available all over Europe. In 1984, the United States Food and Drug Administration approved it for prescription use. Today, they are on the WHO List of Essential Medicines, marking them as effective and safe to use.

NRT: TYPES AND USES

The Nicorette gums were soon in use and helped ease withdrawal symptoms. However, it is still best to consult a doctor before you start taking NRT and it will help you fix the dosage as per your requirement. Generally, the treatment lasts from 12-24 weeks in which a controlled dosage of nicotine is consumed. Since the launch of the Nicorette Gum, many products have been launched and enjoyed good success. They are available as gums, patches, lozenges, inhalers and others. Let's take a look at how one can use them:

Gums:

This is the most common alternative. Gums are easy to chew and last for 20-30 minutes. People can choose the dosage as per their requirements. The tablets come from 1 mg to 4mg. The dosage is dependent on the type of user. It is absorbed through the mouth lining and should not be swallowed. It works on a modified-release dosage, that is, the drug is released slowly and has a longer impact. Also, it is advised to avoid eating any food since it might reduce the effect of the gum. They are generally recommended for 6-12 weeks. The quantity of the gums reduce with time. Some people might find the taste bitter. They might face irritation, changes in saliva production, nausea or headaches. In case they are extreme, it is better to talk to a doctor or reduce the intake.

Lozenges:

They are similar to gums and available over the counter. It is best to manage cravings by not taking more than one lozenge at a time. That said, 9 lozenges a day are adequate. You can reduce the quantity as the cravings reduce.

Nasal sprays:

They are available only as per prescription. The individual is required to spray directly into the nasal membranes. One dose is equal to two sprays. They have the lowest strength (0.5mg- 1 mg). Your expert will help you determine how many doses are needed in a day. It might cause irritation in the nose and throat. Some people also experience a runny nose, slight discomfort like sneezing, coughing. But nothing major!

Patches and Inhalers:

These are transdermal patches and are applied on the skin. Their range varies from 5mg- 52.5 mg. The drug flows into the bloodstream through the skin. They work for 16-24 hours. Similarly inhalers are also available as per prescription. They deliver nicotine directly into your mouth so it can be absorbed through mucus. Many people also go for them to stop smoking cigarettes after developing respiratory illnesses.

NRT products give a satiating feeling while reducing cravings. It works differently for everyone. There is no right time to start therapy. You can take on gums, lozenges or inhalers the moment you choose to stop smoking. They help with the physical dependency. However, with reduced consumption of nicotine, an individual will face some withdrawal symptoms. Don't worry, there are ways to manage them as well. Many people choose to be part of support groups. Hearing other people's stories and struggles inspire them to stick to the path. Given the massive side effects of consuming nicotine, many people are inclined to go for NRT.

ARE YOU THE RIGHT CANDIDATE?

You can opt for NRT, in case if you:

- Feel intense cravings after meals, during breaks, with coffee, while working,
- Start the day with a cigarette (within 5 minutes of waking up),
- Feel the need to smoke during fight or flight scenarios,
- Smoke more than a pack a day,
- Wake up at night to smoke.

NRT doses are decided based on how many cigarettes you consume a day. For example:

Less than 10 cigarettes daily = less than 2 tobacco pouches weekly,

10-20 cigarettes daily = 2-3 tobacco pouches weekly,

1 or more pack of cigarettes = 3 tobacco pouches weekly.

Just a quick reminder: ***NRT is not universal.***

Let's have a quick look at who should not directly jump into this therapy.

- Pregnant women,
- Teenagers,
- Present smokers,
- People who have experienced heart related problems in the past.

The products have small side effects like high saliva production, irritation, headaches, etc. However, when not consumed cautiously, they can lead to some serious problems like nicotine poisoning. Some of the symptoms are hyper salivation, nausea, vomiting and addiction. For pregnant women it can reach the placenta and breast milk, for both active and passive smoking mothers. It puts the fetus at the risk of obesity, hypertension, diabetes, and even ADHD. Hence pregnant women and teenagers are encouraged to opt for behavioural therapy.

But wait…

It is said that nicotine has improved the symptoms of severe depression. If yes, then how? Were we not just discussing in the previous chapter how it destroys dopamine and causes depression? Well, both claims are right. It is both, a bane and a boon when it comes to mental disorders.

A STEP TOWARDS BETTER MENTAL HEALTH

NRT is known to improve neurodegenerative disorders. Nicotine is known as a cognitive enhancer. As we have read in the earlier chapter, it interacts with different parts of the brain and triggers many chemical reactions leading to a functional shift. NRT is being considered to treat many brain disorders. Let,s learn how effective it has been.

Finding a balance: Nicotine helps improve cognitive activities. It has an overall positive impact on working memory and enhances attention. Remember, how after a smoke people think better, how their focus boost up? It does so by changing the synaptic plasticity. Now let's have a look at the behind the scenes. Simply speaking, it activates the signalling pathway by activating protein *CaMKII*. The protein maintains the heart rate, learning, and memory.

It also helps manage disorders like Alzheimer's and Parkinson's. It enhances *protein kinase B Akt* which manages metabolism and cell growth. It activates the Kinase/Akt signalling pathway, enabling cell growth and resilience which helps cope with stress. It also assists in managing Parkinson's disease which is a neurodegenerative disorder that mainly affects movement. Nicotine reduces the production of *Sirtuin 6 (SIRT6)* which manages aging, DNA repair, and manages stress. It also manages metabolism and neuronal health. The overproduction of *SIRT6* can lead to neuronal death. It slows down the progression of the diseases. All in all, nicotine in controlled dosage helps improve the mental state of the patient. In the long term it is fatal, but when used wisely, it still has something to offer.

CONNECTING DOTS: BRAIN & NICOTINE

The primary reason individuals engage in smoking is to feel better or "alleviate stress". There is a high chance that people with neural disorders are smokers or use smoking as a coping mechanism. As per the research, 40-60 percent people dealing with depression are smokers. We have learnt earlier how it triggers dopamine production, creating a feeling of reward. It has shown to reduce depression. One more benefit is its immediate effect. Normal antidepressants take longer to show effects. NRT can prove to be helpful where antidepressants lack. This particularly helps older people. It has been affirmed by brain imaging techniques like fMRI and PET. They track real time activity and help to read how the brain reacts to nicotine. It has been shown that nicotine enhances connectivity between the brain reward regions. Hence, it signals towards a solution for patients struggling with brain disorders.

Nicotine as a treatment has gained increasing relevance over the years. Researchers are also becoming more focused on learning and developing new treatments. This does not mean we can ignore its addictive nature. During NRT, it's very important to manage the registration of the dosage otherwise it can lead to addiction. They also need to be carried under proper supervision. The use of NRT can cause irritation, high blood pressure, and increased heart rate. There have also been cases of hypertension and heart complications. Long term and high use can impair long term synaptic plasticity. Hence teenagers are also advised to refrain from becoming dependent NRT. Only depending on nicotine to deal with depression can lead to further complications. It also poses the risk of dementia. After a time, the effect of reward fades away. Hence it is stressed to join behavioural therapy with NRT.

NRT has been a go to go option for many people. It is an excuse from cigarettes, if not nicotine. Its uses to treat other disorders/diseases continue to be discussed. There are other ways to start your *quit smoking journey* like behavioural therapy. Many individuals can also track their progress on digital apps like Kwit and quitSTART. There are many international support groups. They connect more people and share helpful tips. For example, Action on Smoking and Health is a dedicated autonomous group which raises public awareness on the negative effects of smoking. Joining these community groups gives the individual the support needed to continue their journey of quitting. They are a reminder that you are not alone. There are platfroms and people to support you.

People do know that nicotine harms them. They do know its innumerable long term consequences. It's not that they don't stop because they don't want to. They CAN'T stop since the brain is wired to become addicted to nicotine because of release of dopamine. The constant "urge", the dependence is the reason that people struggle. NRT comes as a saviour in such a situation. It helps to manage this "dependency" by reducing the urge. It's not a one stop solution, but it hints towards the light at the end of the tunnel.

Chapter – 7
A PARADOX

NRT is an effective treatment with a good success rate. However, there is always a lingering risk of addiction that comes with it. For this reason, people like to combine it with a safer option like *Cognitive Behavioural Therapy.* CBT is a long term process which starts from scratch. It is an interconnected approach. It works on the idea that thoughts, emotions, and behaviours are all connected. That means you act based on how you feel. Unfortunately, your thoughts might not always be for the best or do good to you.

Let's try to understand with the hypothesis: **Negative thoughts lead to self destructive behaviours.** How? Well, when one thinks *"I can't get a simple task done, I am good at nothing"*, or *"Bad things always happen to me"*, such thoughts trigger stress, leading to more fear and anxiety. People often look for coping mechanisms to feel short term relief. These mechanisms could be substance abuse like smoking or physical harm. Many people develop eating disorders, go into isolation, or act impulsively. All these actions provide short term dopamine release. It makes one feel better in the moment. But does not solve the core issue - negative thoughts also known as cognitive distortions.

BREAKING THE CYCLE

CBT focuses directly on the issue. It works on reducing or changing the primary thoughts which lead to self destructive behavior. **Aaron T Beck** was the person who developed cognitive therapy. He called these thoughts "*Automatic thoughts*", meaning, the thoughts were not conscious but coming from a space of emotional distress. After the publication of his research, he was referred to as "**The Father of Cognitive Behavioural Therapy.**" It was first developed to help people struggling from depression, PTSD, or anxiety disorders. However, today, it is relevant in treating substance addiction, including smoking.

It is a psychological approach which helps individuals to identify the "WHY"- why does the person feel like smoking? And why is the urge stronger at some specific times? It helps to build willpower to quit and prevent relapse. It helps to manage negative talk which is one big reason pushing people towards addiction. A better self image boosts morale to adopt healthier habits. So how does it work?

CBT is "action oriented". It starts from working on cognitive distortions. These are mainly thoughts and opinions which generally hinder our ability to think clearly. We know that while angry, we often end up speaking things we regret later. Similarly, it believes that cognitive distortions force wrong behaviours which can further lead to many mental disorders.

Does it provide any solution?

Well, yes. Let's have a look at the procedure:

Step 1: Identify Triggering Thoughts

Trigger thoughts are basically "automatic thoughts". They might happen at specific conditions, like when one is feeling angry, irritated, or buzzed. These situations are generally followed by high stress hormones like cortisol and adrenaline. They blur the ability to think rationally. As a result, what the mind craves is for a little comfort, or a feeling of relief. This feeling comes from nicotine and thus the person rushes to smoke. Some of these situations are:

- "Work was hectic, I want a cigarette."
- "I like my coffee with a cigarette."
- "I have had an intense argument, I need a smoke to think clearly. "

These might be different for every individual. CBT identifies these thought patterns and changes them.

Step 2: Coping Strategy

Once you recognise where the trouble is, it is time to fix it. Through CBT, individuals can go for coping strategies which suit them well. Let's take from the examples above:

- After a busy day of work, an individual can look for a good meal, movie, or a sweet treat to help feel relaxed. It helps to boost dopamine.
- During some intense emotions, pause, breathe, and wait for 10 minutes before you light a cigarette. There is a high chance that the craving might go away.

Remember: It may take a while to create these "conscious constructive habits". Have patience as you progress.

Step 3: Changing the Pattern

These refer to the different activities which help change the pattern. They break the cycle of nicotine dependence. It includes:

- Rethinking: It first changes the thoughts which promote such behaviour. It pushes the individual to think positively. For example – "I enjoy coffee without a cigarette too."

- Alternative Action: These include grabbing a snack or having water, instead of a smoke.
- Self counselling: Individual has to consciously talk to himself out of the urge. One might not have an alternative option at all times. In these moments, it is important to remind ourselves – "**Smoking is not the solution.**"

Step 4: Progress

The last step involves keeping up with the above activities. During situations like social gathering, or periods of high stress, there is a high chance the person might give into temptation. It is important to rely on trusted people who can help you keep control your need to smoke.

As mentioned, it is a long term solution that takes a long time to take effect. But how long? Well, it depends how deep you are into the loop. Generally people take about 5-10 sessions. It can extend in case of a relapse. The sessions are mainly decided by:

- The duration,
- Severity of the symptoms,
- Your environment,
- Stress,
- Any other existing medical condition.

WHO IS THE RIGHT THERAPIST FOR YOU?

CBT requires some background research. Remember it is a "*talk therapy*". Hence it becomes important that you reach out to the right therapist/counsellor. Now how do you decide?

- Well, have a quick look at their credentials. You can look for their educational qualifications (Bachelors and Masters degree is mandatory in India). This will help you to build trust.
- You can also check if their description matches your needs. Ensure that your therapist has a licence from the state to practise. This will further give them credibility.
- You can have a call with them to know about their expertise. You can consult specifically your symptoms, and any other disorder which you might be struggling with.

Quitting nicotine might feel like a big step but CBT professionals make your journey easier. The sessions are carried out one on one. You can also join self help groups and interact with a wider crowd. The primary thing is to build trust. If you feel you are not ready for CBT, you can confide in a friend or a family member.

Is CBT enough?

Heavy smokers often feel CBT is not enough for them. Hence they opt for **Partial Agonists.** These are medicinal drugs. As the name suggests, they produce half the effect. Some of the examples are: *buprenorphine, buspirone, aripiprazole.* They stimulate nAChRs, but the effect is less than the original dose. It initiates a slight dopamine release. As a result, it helps reduce cravings and manages withdrawal symptoms. At the same time, it mimics dopamine and controls the effects of smoking.

Some of the medications to look up:

Varenicline is the most popular and easily available. It is considered THE BEST for smoking cessation. It is more effective than NRT gums and patches. It is a 12 week course which is available on prescription. In the US it is marketed as *Chantix* and outside as *Champix*. They directly target the nicotine receptors in the brain. It works in two primary ways:

It binds to the a4b3 receptors in the brain which play a key role in the reward system. This is where dopamine is released from. Unlike nicotine, it doesn't fully activate them. It slightly stimulates them leading to a small release of dopamine. This way, it helps manage the withdrawal symptoms. Second, it prevents nicotine from binding to the receptors. Hence, people fail to feel the pleasure that comes from smoking. This helps to reduce cravings.

People can also go for **Cytisine** which works similarly to varenicline. It is specific to Eastern Europe and is not available worldwide. Comparatively, it is much cheaper. Individuals might feel nausea, headaches, or mood swings when using it. It is also advised that people with mental health disorders refrain from taking these medicines without consultation.

COMPLETE BLOCKAGE

Another variety of Antagonists that absolutely stop the effect of nicotine are also available. They come in a 12-week course available on prescription. In a few cases, the timeline is extended, especially if there is a danger of relapse. Some of the main medications under this category are listed here.

Bupropion was first created as an antidepressant and sold as *Wellbutrin.* Later, it was discovered that it can help with reducing smoking effects. Then it was marketed as *Zyban*. It primarily modifies the neurotransmitters. That means it makes an impact on how your brain communicates. It is classified as an Norepinephrine Reuptake Inhibitor (NDRI). Meaning? It increases dopamine and norepinephrine. Being an antagonist, it blocks nicotine from binding to these receptors. Hence, the nicotine does not release any dopamine.

Since quitting nicotine leads to low levels of dopamine, hence it mimics nicotine's effects and helps to manage withdrawal symptoms. It is especially good for people who have a history of depression or anxiety. It does not cause weight gain, bad gut health, or drowsiness which is an issue with other antidepressants. This makes it a perfect fit.

Mecamylamine is another antagonist. It stops nicotine induced dopamine release. This helps to reduce the addictive effects. It is preferred in combination with nicotine replacement therapy. People might face issues like dry mouth, increased heart rate or insomnia.

BEST OF BOTH

But, is it possible to have the best of both therapies?

Yes. For those, who need both counselling and medications, the option of **Combination Therapy** is available. It combines two or more treatments. It increases the chance of quitting smoking. Generally it helps heavy smokers who have a history of depression. Combination therapy provides flexibility and helps people with heavy smoking and mental health conditions. The combination is:

Pharmacological Medicines + Behavioural Therapy.

That means combining NRT/medicines with counselling. There are a couple of options:

- Trying different forms of NRT like using patches with gums for both immediate and long term hits.
- Combining NRT and prescription medications. Like using patches/gums with bupropion. It helps reduce cravings while maintaining dopamine and norepinephrine levels.
- Combining varenicline and bupropion. Here the former blocks nicotine's effects while the latter manages the dopamine levels.
- Last is CBT and NRT - using patches and counselling. It helps to maintain both physical health and mental health.

Nicotine never fails to surprise us. It is a paradox - both the addiction and its solution. NRT is a treatment which uses small doses of nicotine. For people who want to embrace an absolutely nicotine free life, CBT is a good option. It might take longer and is especially good for people who are light smokers. People can, of course, rely on pharmacological aid like NRT and partial agonists. Combination therapy on the other hand gives one the option to end addiction and build good will power. CBT has a success rate of 60-75 percent.

After the sessions, many people overcome their addiction and mood disorders.

For those inclined towards pharmacological medicines like antagonists, consult your doctor. They will help you schedule the doses. Also, teenagers, pregnant women, or heart patients are advised to not take medicines without consultation. They can lead to serious health effects including nicotine poisoning.

Well, now you know that quitting nicotine can be a pleasant journey with the right help. Recovery will help you have more say over your mind and body. It is time to abandon short term dopamine which fools your brain.

Let's start once again, with the right help, towards a healthier life.

Chapter - 8
TEENAGERS AND THERAPY

There is a popular saying: An adolescent brain develops till **25** years of age. Every experience, event, activity, and habit has a profound impact on building the brain. Similarly, substance use like alcohol exposure, drugs, or nicotine directly shapes neural connections. The number of teenagers who smoke between the age of 13-15 is alarming. Almost **50 million** teenagers are engaged in some form of nicotine consumption. This huge population is a constant worry. Almost 60 percent of this population tries to quit, but only 5 percent use NRT. Feels surprising since NRT is the most affordable and least taxing way to quit. Its side effects could be a possible reason that most "young adolescents" refrain from using it. It might suppress your cravings for the time being but fails to build long-term resilience. Though NRT products are not as addictive, the risk is always there. Hence, it is not the preferred therapy for youth. So, do young adolescents have no way out?

Let's first learn WHY we can not use NRT when it comes to teenagers.

Let's start with the "brain" of a teenager, which is still under development. From our earlier chapters, we know that nicotine weakens neural connections. Its consumption in teenagers poses risk to brain development. NRT helps them quit smoking. However, the chances of relapse and addiction are higher. In the long term, we see side effects like cognitive impairment, impact on neural circuits, struggle in decision making, and chances of addiction.

These changes are not visible initially. Instead, initially, we experience the thrill of it all. But a lot starts to happen inside your brain: The prefrontal cortex, a highly important part of the brain, matures till a later stage in life. It is located right behind your forehead and handles decision-making, impulse control, and reasoning. Maybe that's why the saying goes big forehead means big brains. For example, the urge to have a sweet, go on a trip impulsively, build a habit, are all managed by the prefrontal cortex. Till its maturation, it is sensitive and adapts quickly to new habits and environments. Sadly, nicotine is no exception. What feels like a "little fun" can pose a major risk later.

THE STORY OF THE FIRST "PUFF"

Statistics say that the first "hit" is experienced between 16 and 20 years of age. Around 60 percent of teen smokers end up with an addiction. Initially, we think *"It's no biggie, I can quit anytime."* What the teenager does not realise is that with every puff the brain is becoming wired to nicotine.

But how is it any different from a mature, developed brain?

Adolescence is the age when we feel most energised and eager to try new things. It is the age to "take risks" and "try it all". This is also the time when your brain is undergoing major changes like puberty or sexual maturation. During this time, every action defines the brain's plasticity. Your brain is continuously adapting to what you do, see and learn during these years.

When you use nicotine regularly, the brain signal pathway changes. As a result, the brain feels foggy and confused. It becomes hard to function without that "morning" cigarette. This, right here, shows dependency. The signal pathway is used to feel the "hit" to work efficiently. These are the changes a person might feel in a couple of months. And, in the long term, poor decisions, inability to think rationally, memory loss, weak attention span, poor emotional regulation and movement are some of the concerning issues.

Let's understand how nicotine moulds your prefrontal cortex connections. The prefrontal cortex is located in the frontal lobe - that means right behind your forehead and extends towards the temples. It is the largest lobe. It bears the brunt of major accidents and experiences. From decision-making to handling traumatic injuries, the prefrontal cortex does it all. How you decide if a situation is risky, solve a problem, or react to a stressful event is dependent on it. It is backed by a strong neural network to work effectively. A good signal system keeps it updated with all and assists to take a decision. In the absence of neurotransmitter signalling, PFC has trouble making decisions.

A DOPAMINE CRISIS

Nicotine influences two major signal systems, *dopaminergic* and *cholinergic* systems, confusing the brain. With unclear direction, the prefrontal cortex, that is the forebrain starts to lag. Initially, it might be just forgetting to pack your charger, but later on, it can turn into a disorder like Alzheimer's.

What do dopaminergic and cholinergic pathways do that is so important?

Nicotine hijacks your dopaminergic system, the unit which handles your happy hormones and mood. It immediately boosts dopamine levels. It gives the feeling of thrill, happiness or light-heartedness. You must recall from early chapters that dopamine is a hormone and a neurotransmitter. There are other activities too which influence this pathway like socialising, eating good food, exercising, or watching a movie. Humans, by default, like to enjoy these experiences of reward and happiness. The brain locates the source of happiness, in this case, it is nicotine. It signals the prefrontal cortex to consume more nicotine. With repetition of this process, the brain plasticity is changed. Now, the highest level of dopamine it can feel is through nicotine, leading to dependence. Once your signalling pathway is used to dopamine, its "craving" is increased. There is a constant urge to "smoke" to feel relaxed.

Simply put, nicotine takes over the dopaminergic pathways. Your brain is no longer making the final call. The brain falls prey to poor thinking and decision-making. As a result, teenagers often give in to the temptation and act impulsively. Comparatively, they have a more sensitive dopamine system. Hence, the overall impact is amplified, increasing the risk of addiction and other health consequences.

Nicotine damage is both physiological and psychological. It disturbs the signalling pathway which in turn disturbs cognitive activities. Your cholinergic system maintains cognitive activities like learning and memory. In an ideal case, the system helps the brain focus, making space for new information. It leads to habits like self-control, focus and rational decision making.

The period of adolescence is marked by synaptic pruning. It's like a filtering process. It’s the survival of the fittest. The prefrontal cortex removes the weaker connections, holding onto the stronger ones. These connections define your interests. The more a particular activity is repeated the stronger the brain strands become. The pruning process ensures that only useful neural networks remain. In this way, it clears space, allowing space for new learning.

Now nicotine enters the brain. It mimics acetylcholine, stimulating nAChRs in the prefrontal cortex. The normal process of filtering neurons is disturbed. The brain receives confused signals. This interferes with the neural connections. The person ends up experiencing weak focus. The brain’s organisation is disturbed causing weaker and poorer connections. Isn’t it amusing how a smoke puff can damage our brains?

& THE LORE GOES ON…

Dopaminergic and cholinergic pathways are severely influenced as a result of smoking, but that’s not the end of it. Our brains have many small parts, each having their own role. In a young developing brain, nicotine immediately influences:

- the ventral striatum stimulating high reward carvings,
- and the dorsolateral prefrontal cortex which is still under development.

Even though the ventral striatum tries to manage cravings, because of an underdeveloped prefrontal cortex, it fails. The hippocampus region is also disturbed which manages memory retention.

Over time there is a change in the consumption pattern as well. 15.5 percent of the youth today vape, while 80 percent prefer cigarettes. Many adolescents today are subjected to stress from an early age. They find cigarettes as a means of relaxation. In their daily lives, they experience emotional dysregulation. Mental anxieties like mood swings, depression, and brain fog are increasing. The brain feels cluttered because the pruning process gets hindered.

Its decision making power is reduced. It can not decide which neuron to filter out. Hence there is so much going on and you feel spaced out.

The risk association with nicotine and NRT are higher for a young adolescent. It is mainly because of their developing brain. The chance of relapse and addiction is also higher. There have been studies that show images of exact processes happening inside the brain. Techniques like Positron Emission Tomography (PET) and Functional Magnetic Resonance Imaging (fMRI) provide valuable insights. These studies help to map addiction, cognitive impairment, and withdrawal effects.

DEVELOPMENT TIMELINE

Before the development of these studies, earlier methods existed and testing was done primarily on animals. Let us look at how far we have come in our understanding of the issue.

The 1950s: Scientists confirmed nicotine leads to better moods.

1970:s nAChRs were discovered. It was confirmed that nicotine mimics the acetylcholine neurotransmitter.

1980s: The mesolimbic pathway was established.

Positron Emission Tomography (PET) Studies

PET was discovered by **Edward J Hoffman** and **Michael E Phelps**. It creates 3D images and can be combined with a CT scan to produce more detailed images. It tracks down neurotransmitter changes.

Mechanism: It studies the effect of nicotine on the brain through radiation. It uses a radiolabeled dopamine racer. A radiotracer is injected into your arms. In most cases, it is fluorodeoxyglucose (FDG). It is similar to the glucose produced in our bodies. The areas studied are the striatum and nucleus accumbens. This helps track addictive behaviour. It shows changes in receptors in different parts of the brain like the prefrontal cortex, and hippocampus.

Result: The results showed dependence, high alertness, and metabolic activity. When nicotine is dropped, there is fatigue, brain fog, and difficulty in focusing.

Functional Magnetic Resonance Imaging (fMRI)

fMRI was developed by **Seiji Ogawa**. It is very effective since it gives real-time insights. It tells you exactly what is going on inside your brain. By checking the blood flow, one learns how one action leads another in the brain. It helps us to know how well a medical drug works and how it interacts with the blood-brain barrier.

Our brain needs oxygen to function well. Whenever there is an increased activity in any neuron, the oxygen-rich blood level is increased. fMRI scanner catches this change.

Mechanism: Oxygenated hemoglobin does not cause any changes in the magnetic fields. The fMRI signals remain high. On the other hand, deoxygenated hemoglobin causes disturbance in magnetic fields leading to decreased signals. As active parts of the brain receive more oxygen than they use there is an increase in oxygenated blood. These results are known as oxygen level-dependent signals (BOLD).

The whole process happens over a period of time. It is known as **Hemodynamic Response Function.** It happens in three stages:

- Initial dip: A weak signal. More oxygen consumption by neurons.
- Peak response: This is the phase where more blood is delivered than needed. It results in a strong fMRI signal.
- Post-Stimulus Undershoot: The blood retreats to baseline causing a dip.

Result: fMRI shows better working memory and cognitive attention when nicotine is consumed. We also see changes in the default mode network (DMN). The area appears weak, struggling to take decisions. Lastly, we have the amygdala which shows reduced activity. The amygdala reacts to stress or distressed emotions. Hence, for a short while, the negative thoughts are reduced, giving the feeling of relaxation.

PET and fMRI are effective techniques to map down changes. When using nicotine, the images show the same changes: better working attention, relaxation, reduced negative thoughts, and weaker connections. For a safe recovery and the least damage to brain development, teenagers are not recommended NRT. But there are options like CBT which are an effective way to quit smoking. CBT offers long-term recovery without building any dependence. It also helps build a supportive environment.

Quitting smoking is the right thing to do, but it is important to do it correctly. It might seem tough at the present, but it's possible. Do the right thing, and do it the right way. In the end, you will thank yourself for making a tough but healthy decision.

Chapter - 9
WOULD YOU LIKE SOME COFFEE?

Throughout history, humans have been using many substances to feel that magical *"hit"*. Many natural compounds give a soothing feeling, taking us to cloud nine. We know nicotine is one such stimulant. Its benefits have been known for long. But it is not the ONLY stimulant. There is another drug which produces similar effects. We have been using it every day to energise our mornings. Yes, You got it right - **Caffeine**.

Caffeine is widely consumed around the globe. The "coffee industry" is out there and progressing day by day. It has a long and interesting history. Discovered in Ethiopia in 850 A.D, it is used in many beverages with tea and coffee being the most popular ones. It became known to the wider world in the 15th and 16th centuries when the English started consuming it. However, its first usage can be traced back to the Tang dynasty in 600 AD. In 1819, Friedlieb Ferdinand Runge isolated and named the compound. Today, it is part of every household and today's work culture functions entirely on coffee cups. Coffee, we can see, has travelled a long way.

A BRIEF BACKGROUND CHECK

Caffeine is a white organic alkaloid found in plants native to South America, East Asia, and Africa.

Fun Fact: It is naturally produced in plants as a defence mechanism. Caffeine has proven to affect the behaviour of warm bugs found in plants which disturb their growth. We will learn how it affects the human brain. You already know it keeps you up and alert, but only when consumed in the right amount. When consumed in its natural form it can turn lethal. One tablespoon of natural powered caffeine equals about 84 mugs of coffee. Its side effects are visible in our daily lives, like dehydration, poor gut health, insomnia, irritation and more.

The number of drinks that have caffeine will surprise you. Coffee, tea, cocoa, kola nut, chewing gum, and of course energy drinks. Let's quickly go through the list of contents:

COFFEE

No household is unfamiliar with coffee's aroma and its variety. From Americano to instant coffee, all coffee comes from coffee beans. The effect coffee has on you varies depending on the quality of the beans. For instance, an Arabica bean contains around 2 mg of caffeine, Robusta 3 mg, and Liberica just 1 mg. The brewing method further determines how strong the effect of the stimulant is. For instance, one cup of filtered coffee has 85 mg of caffeine, one cup of instant coffee has 65 mg, and one cup of an espresso shot has 60 mg of caffeine.

Hence, coffee has a good amount of caffeine which helps fight drowsiness, gives a dopamine rush, and is a perfect stimulant. However, one should be careful as it can lead to irritation and headaches.

TEA

Tea is a widely popular beverage, especially in Asia. It comes from the *Camellia sinensis* plant. It also contains caffeine but is not as strong as coffee. Black tea is the strongest and contains the most caffeine. Its effect depends on how well the tea leaves have been boiled/brewed. The market today sees an increased potential for herbal tea, which is caffeine-free.

CHOCOLATE

Everybody loves a sugar rush! But chocolate isn't only sweet. It also contains caffeine. The amount is not too high, hence one does not feel the effect for long. But all of us can confirm feeling cheery immediately after having chocolate. It can be because of the sugar rush or caffeine from the cocoa beans. Chocolate contains only 5 per cent caffeine.

ENERGY DRINKS

Energy drinks are growing in popularity. Caffeinated drinks like Coca-Cola have enjoyed glorious profits. For health reasons, there has been an increasing demand for non-caffeinated drinks like Sprite. But where does the caffeine in these drinks come from - beans, extract, or some plant?

Well, the primary ingredient used is the the extract of kola nuts containing caffeine. There is a ban on the use of Kola nuts in America. However, in India, it is still used for production of some caffeinated beverages. The alternative was found in soda. It slowly progressed to artificially produced caffeine known as synthetic caffeine. Both have similar chemical properties. The only difference is the absorption process. Synthetic caffeine gets absorbed more quickly and hence gives an immediate energy rush.

CAFFIENE DEPENDENCY: REAL BUT OVERLOOKED

There is a long debate over the nature of caffeine. Research has proven that caffeine consumption shoots up cortisol and adrenaline levels. When consumed mindfully, it makes you feel refreshed. When consumed in high doses, it can make one feel anxious and give trouble while sleeping.

Yes, it is possible to develop a caffeine addiction. Most people are not aware of it but they are dependent on caffeine. Generally, one feels high mental and physical energy within 10-30 minutes of consuming caffeine.

Caffeine dependency is real. It is hard to pinpoint the exact number, but the addiction rate is at 35 percent. It might not hit you immediately, but slowly and surely it shows up. Hence when you suddenly stop consuming caffeine, there is a restlessness. It is not severe. Rather, it feels like something is missing which can get you going. It's a common complaint among elder females who are dependent on caffeine. They often complain about headaches in the morning till they have their *dear tea*. This right here is a withdrawal symptom. Since coffee has the highest caffeine concentration amongst beverages, people have high dependency and struggle to cope without it. Some of the symptoms experienced are irritation, anxiety, fatigue, brain fog, and lesser dopamine.

Very similar to nicotine, right? If we look closely, there is a similarity in dependence patterns for caffeine and nicotine. It is because they impact the same neural pathway.

But, what does it mean?

Both caffeine and nicotine increase the neurotransmitter activity leading to more alertness, attention, and better cognitive experience. They both influence the dopamine-reward system making us feel motivated. However there are some differences which makes caffeine a safer option.

The first difference is in the dopaminergic pathway. In the last chapter, we saw that dopaminergic is the brain's reward pathway. As we know nicotine combines with nAChRs which trigger dopamine release and caffeine blocks the adenosine A2 receptors increasing dopamine. But comparatively, the effect is less than nicotine. This primary difference makes nicotine more addictive, because of the strong rewarding effect.

The second difference that has been noticed is in the cholinergic pathway. This pathway maintains cognitive activities and alertness. Nicotine acts as an *agonist* and stimulates neural activity. It is observed by an increase in the release of acetylcholine. Hence, we see immediate results like better attention, working memory, and motivation. Caffeine blocks the adenosine A1 receptor which prevents drowsiness and clears brain fog. Adenosine is a naturally occurring compound. It manages your sleep, wakefulness, and other crucial brain activities. When it binds to the brain receptors, it leads to drowsiness and slow neural activity. Caffeine blocks these receptors. It is capable of affecting all 4 types of adenosine receptors: A1, A2A, A2B, and A3.

The third similarity is better cognitive activity and attention span. Even though both are stimulants, their effects vary. Nicotine improves working memory and reaction time. However, relying on it reduces memory span in the long term. Caffeine improves alertness. Its dependence does not cause any long-term cognitive damage. It is because unlike nicotine, it does not cause any changes in brain plasticity.

INTRODUCING AMPHETAMINES

There is one more stimulant - Amphetamines. Unlike caffeine and nicotine, it is not naturally occurring. It is a synthetic stimulant drug. *Adderall, Dexedrine,* and *Vyvanse* are some drugs that contain Amphetamines. They heavily affect the central nervous system.

So, how are Amphetamines produced?

Technically speaking, Amphetamines are derivates of phenylisopropylamine. It was first made in 1887 by Lazâr Edeleanu and he was the one who named it phenylisopropylamine. However, its stimulant properties were discovered in 1927 by Gordon Alles. Post that, it was marketed by many companies for decongestion. Slowly, it was prescribed for many medical conditions like narcolepsy, obesity, and blood pressure. After many regulations, today, it is used for treating ADHD, narcolepsy, and eating disorders.

It may come as a surprise to you how long amphetamines have been in use. From being used by soldiers in WW2 for alertness, to treating medical conditions like sleeping and eating disorders, to being part of mod culture in the UK for partying all night. It has been under a lot of scrutiny because of its severe addictive nature. It has been proven that long-term use causes detrimental effects like anxiety, paranoia, hallucinations and more.

How does it affect the human brain?

We will understand this process in 5 easy steps:

- It binds with the transporter protein, Monoamine.
- It interacts with Dopamine Transporter (DAT) and boosts dopamine levels.
- It interacts with Norepinephrine Transporter (NET) and boosts norepinephrine levels. This causes an increase in alertness and attention.
- With the transporter, it gets inside the neurons, interfering with the synapses.
- It also boosts up neurotransmitters prolonging the effect.

Hence, its impact is pretty visible:

- Very high dopamine levels, giving a euphoric feeling leading to an addictive nature and
- Higher attention level because of the high level of norepinephrine.

So, is it any better than caffeine or nicotine? Well, all the three stimulants build dependency and lead to one or other side effects. A comparative summary will help us more:

Primary Action

Nicotine: Influences nACHhRs leading to dopamine release.

Caffeine: Blocks adenosine receptors causing wakefulness.

Amphetamines: Influences DAT and NET leading to an increase in dopamine and norepinephrine levels.

Effect on Brain

Nicotine: It stimulates the reward and cognitive pathway. This leads to addiction.

Caffeine: Boost energy levels without directly influencing dopamine levels. Hence, there is no risk of addiction.

Amphetamines: Releases high levels of dopamine for a longer time, creating a feeling of euphoria. It has a severe risk of drug addiction.

Cognitive Effects

Nicotine: Better working memory in the short term. Consistent use in the long term can cause both psychological and physiological impairment.

Caffeine: It increases focus and attention, reducing fatigue. It has no long-term health risk.

Amphetamines: It is known for improving attention and cognitive performance. It is useful in treating ADHD.

Health Risk

Nicotine: There is a risk of respiratory and cardiovascular diseases and cancer.

Caffeine: When consumed in high doses it leads to insomnia, heart palpitations, and anxiety.

Amphetamines: It has severe withdrawal symptoms like cardiac issues, psychosis and more.

CROSS ADDICTION: WHICH ONE TO PICK?

Based on the above, we can not say one stimulant is better than the other. Caffeine, when consumed as a beverage like coffee/tea is good and risk-free. Whereas nicotine when consumed through cigarettes, causes health damage but also boosts current working memory. The last is Amphetamines, which is a crucial medical drug in treating ADHD, otherwise, it can lead to fatal damage. We can classify their usage depending on their addiction levels, where caffeine has the least, followed by nicotine and then Amphetamines.

Individuals can consume two or all three stimulants simultaneously. Cross-addiction is very common, where one person quits one stimulant but develops a dependency on another. This is seen most when a person is trying to quit smoking, and they start relying on coffee. Many like to take nicotine and caffeine together, where one boosts the appetite for the other. People taking Amphetamines depend on nicotine since the effect produced is similar. Hence, cross addiction happens continuously, as per individual differences. However, all three stimulants come with their troubling withdrawal symptoms:

Nicotine: Anxiety, difficulty in concentrating, irritation, cravings, and poor cognition function.

Caffeine: Drowsiness, fatigue, haedches.

Amphetamines: Fatigue, intense cravings, high cognitive impairment, fatigue, and depression.

Nicotine, caffeine and Amphetamines are popular stimulants. They are known for their medical use, especially in treating neurodegenerative diseases. However, when used without proper medical guidance, they can prove to be extremely addictive and fatal. From their consumption to consequences, we can see the differences. Hence, use your brain to feed it the right substance which keeps it safe and sound. As long as the dosage is under safe limits, you will sail through.

Chapter – 10
GENE POLYMORPHISM

We see many people around us, who, despite leading a healthy lifestyle end up with serious illnesses. They are physically active, do not indulge in substance use and yet! They are seen struggling with health issues like COPD, cancers or psychological illnesses like depression. The reason is that our health is not dependent only on external factors. Following a healthy routine will definitly be a bonus. But it does not guarantee that you don't become prone to illnesses. Remember, we come from a long lineage of ancestors. Their health also has a role in defining our health. How? Easy, through the law of inheritance! One does not just look like their parents - they share common interests and habits too. If either of the parents has indulged in substance use, there is a high chance that it will impact the baby. That's why during and before pregnancy, parents are advised to stop consuming substances including nicotine and caffeine as it might affect the health of the infant.

Interesting, right?

MAKING OF DNA

Our bodies are made of tissues which are made of millions of cells. Each cell contains a nucleus. In turn, every cell contains our defining particle: the DNA molecule. The first life cells are formed from both parents' reproductive cells: sperm and ovum. The health of the sperm and ovum determine the health of the infant. Nicotine has the potential to change the component of your DNA which passes down to the DNA of the infant.

How does it happen?

As we know, nicotine binds with nicotinic acetylcholine receptors in the central and peripheral nervous systems. It influences mood and causes addictive behaviors. But it doesn't stop there. It also alters the gene containing nACHr subunits. Yes, it really goes deep. This leads to variations in the DNA sequence. It directly interferences with particulars which deals with nicotine dependence. Basically, it gets them used to reacting to nicotine. This process of causing variations in the gene is known as *Genetic Polymorphism*. It primarily happens in two subunits namely:

CHRNA5: This gene has been the subject of much research. It encodes the alpha5 subunit, containing *D398N*. Enough with long names, let's see what it does. It causes changes in ion channels and impacts how nicotine binds with the receptors. Simply speaking, in the long term, it changes the neurotransmitter release, which changes the reward mechanism. A variation in this gene leads to changes in nicotine dependence or how your body interacts with it. It is also associated with handling nicotine addiction, lung cancer, and COPD.

CHRNA3 and **CHRNB4** encode alpha3 and beta4 subunits. They share the same chromosomal region as CHRNA5 and follow a similar trajectory. Variations in these genes lead to changes in neurotransmitter activity.

These two changes were related to the protein nAChRs which lead to the release of neurotransmitters causing reward and pleasure. But they are not the only victims!

Nicotine Metabolism Enzyme, also known as **CYP2A6,** is responsible for the breakdown of nicotine in the liver. It is responsible for converting nicotine into cotinine. Variations in CYP2A6 can lead to changes in enzyme activity. That means it directly influences how long your body sustains nicotine. The possible changes are:

- Reduced Activity: As the name suggests, this variation slows down nicotine metabolism. The slower it breaks, the longer nicotine stays in the blood. Hence, as a result, your body has longer nicotine exposure. It might reduce cravings but the exposure is increased.
- Increased Activity: Similarly, this variation can also increase nicotine metabolism. It incites individuals to smoke more since the effect is short lived. It increases cravings and the risk of addiction.

These variations are tiny. However, they play an important role in managing nicotine cravings. They have a direct role in how an individual adapts to nicotine. The study of Gene Polymorphism is crucial. It can assist health experts in creating better treatments. We can predict behavious and target points. Hence it offers the possibility to map clear solutions.

IS A BAD GENE THE END?

Before forming any misconceptions, please note that a simple variation in the gene is not enough to make you or anyone else a smoker. These variations simply show a slightly increased chance of nicotine dependence. This change is also because their bodies process nicotine differently, increasing the exposure or the craving. The variations have their own role, but it wouldn't be fair to use them as an excuse to pursue smoking.

The variations can also happen in Dopamine Beta-Hydroxylase (DBH) and Catechol-O-Methyltransferase (COMT) genes present in the dopaminergic pathway. These genes handle a variety of functions. The first is the regulation of dopamine, followed by metabolism, and keeping the chemical balance of the brain in control. Variations in these genes have a direct impact on reward and addiction behaviours. A look into the functioning of these genes will help our understanding more.

Dopamine Beta-Hydroxylase (DBH): This gene is responsible for converting dopamine into norepinephrine. These are both hormones and neurotransmitters, handling many physiological activities. The human brain needs a chemical balance to function properly. Hence, this conversion of dopamine to norepinephrine is crucial. It keeps the balance. A change in DBH functions means change in hormones levels. The result is increased or decreased DBH activity.

Decreased activity means slow conversion causing the dopamine levels to increase. With high dopamine, the feeling of pleasure also increases. This in turn leads to nicotine dependency. Conversely, increased activity means fast conversion. This lowers dopamine levels, reducing the rewarding effects. It reduces exposure but also leads to more cravings to feel the desired hit. Hence, the variations in genes regulate the hormone and neurotransmitter levels. Both are important in regulating the chemical balance of the brain.

The same happens with Catechol-O-Methyltransferase (COMT). It is an enzyme that is responsible for the breakdown of catecholamines/neurotransmitters. It also regulates dopamine by transferring a methyl group to them. This process is crucial in regulating the level of dopamine. It especially influences prefrontal control activity. Its variation or gene polymorphism is known as Val158Met.

Hard to understand? Here is a simple way to understand this: Basically, this variation regulates how quickly the dopamine breaks down. For instance:

- Val Genotype is associated with higher COMT activity. As a result, it leads to quick dopamine degradation.
- Met Genotype is associated with lower COMT activity. As a result dopamine degradation slows down making dopamine more available.

Another polymorphism that influences nicotine behaviours are **DRD2** genes. They encode the D2 subtype of the dopamine receptor. This has a central role in maintaining the dopamine effect. Hence, it regulates the reward feeling. So how is it different from the other polymorphism?

Well, DR receptors are found in the mesolimbic pathway. These receptors are associated with maintaining feelings of reward. These receptors are activated by dopamine release which in turn increases pleasure. A variation in this gene directly influences pleasure. Its two variants are:

- **Taq1A** Polymorphism: It is located near the ANKK1 gene adjacent to DRD2. It affects the density of D2 receptors. It has two alleles known as A1 and A2. The A2 allele maintains normal receptor levels. People who carry the A1 allele are bound to experience a slow dopaminergic response, meaning a slow hit. This pushes them to consume more nicotine to experience the desired state of pleasure. Hence, it increases the risk of dependence.

- **C957T** Polymorphism. Its variation is known as 957T. It has an impact on dopamine signalling efficiency.

It is hard to pinpoint the exact number of people who carry these alleles and have smoking dependence. However, research has proved that variations in DRD2 genes change the functioning of these receptors. In return, it confuses the dopamine signals. In the same way, people who carry the A1 or 957T allele experience reduced levels of dopamine activity. They need to have a high intake of nicotine to feel the same pleasure. This mostly ends up in them developing dependence.

A QUICK UPDATE ON BRAIN ACTIVITY

Summarising it, here is what happens when people with gene polymorphism consume nicotine:

Nicotine Intake: It stimulates nicotinic acetylcholine receptors. It is marked by the release of dopamine in the brain's reward pathways.

Dopamine Levels: The neurotransmitter receptors increase the level of dopamine release leading to increased feeling of reward and pleasure. It is important to maintain dopamine levels, which happens through enzyme regulation.

- DBH: It converts dopamine into norepinephrine and maintains the availability of dopamine.

- COMT: It degrades dopamine maintaining dopamine levels.

Addiction Potential: Changes in the normal funcitoning of neurotransmitters have some impact. In case of the above, our body gets wired to feeling pleasure through nicotine. In other words, it gets "addicted" to taking nicotine.

Once, its inside the human body, it affects many functions. To sum it up, we have three main components which are affected:

- **Neurotransmitters**: It concerns dopamine and norepinephrine. Variations affect their production, release, and degradation. It leads to changes in the availability of neurotransmitters. It has a direct impact on rewarding behaviours. Hence, the chances of a person adapting to addiction are dependent on neurotransmitter activity.
- **Receptor Response:** A change in receptor structure influences how nicotine interacts inside the body. It influences decision making, impulse control, and more.
- **Metabolic Rate:** It describes how quickly nicotine breaks down and is removed from the body. It directly influences the amount of nicotine one person consumes to maintain a pleasurable feeling.

GENE VARIATIONS: NOT THE FINAL VEDICT

Not everybody who uses nicotine develops these variations. It is dependent on inheritance patterns, environmental factors, migration patterns and more. Environment too affects nicotine use. Similarly, some groups of people have an ancestry of nicotine. Hence, there is a high chance of occurrence of gene variations in these populations. The percentage of recurring frequency also varies on other factors. For instance, the D398N allele has a frequency of 35 percent in European descent, whereas in the African-American population it is 5 percent. Hence, it does not develop evenly in people and across different populations.

This knowledge of gene variations and addiction patterns has helped in cessation therapies. The genetic history of a person can help with better treatment approaches. Hence, there is no need to be afraid of these genes. They have contributed a lot to pharmacogenetics where a simple gene test can let you know which medicine will work best for the patient.

Addiction patterns are not limited to external factors. Your genes have a major role to play in it. With the advent of better medical facilities, we can hope to create better cessation therapies. Knowledge about them only betters the chances of suitable treatment. They are different, not dangerous. And a healthy lifestyle comes with no regrets!

Chapter – 11
A CALL FOR GLOBAL EFFORT

By now, you know everything about nicotine, from its consumption to its consequences. We have talked about what nicotine is, how it's produced, consumed, and its side effects. We read about a number of therapies like CBT, NRT, and gene therapy, which can help people cope with their addiction.

Nicotine addiction has become a global issue. Researchers from all over the world are talking about it. It poses a threat to both health and productivity. Hence, researchers have been digging into finding more about its functioning in regard to the human body. The better we know it, the better we can handle it.

The centre of curiosity now are Nicotinic Acetylcholine Receptors. They are the hot topic of discussion, since they are the first to meet nicotine inside the body. We have learned that nicotine combines with them. But did you know that the nAChR receptor is also made up of various subunits?

BREAKING DOWN THE RECEPTORS

Yes, the receptor has various subtypes. When nicotine binds to nACHRs, it specifically binds to the subunits. With the advent of better technologies, we can study their functions and changes. Let's start with two important subtypes:

a4b2 and a7: a4b2 is directly associated with nicotine addiction. It has a high liking for nicotine compounds.

Humans are not the only ones with this receptor subtype. It is found in the brains of several mammals. While a4b2 manages the chances of addiction, a7 changes how your brain adapts to nicotine. Subunit a7 changes the neural wiring. A change in brain synapticity means a change in decision-making and managing addiction patterns.

a5 Subunit Variants: They directly influence the function of the nAChR receptors. Since they interfere with the receptor activity, they also manage nicotine dependence. As seen in the previous chapters, gene variations define nicotine addiction and are an important point of study.

Research has shown us the various stages of the nAChR receptors. We can see it resting or inactive, activated or open, and desensitised. A receptor becomes desentisided depending on its ligand binding. Binding here refers to the interaction between nicotine and certain amino acids. It tells the location its influence on receptor activity.

The whole process looks like this: During the activation process, there is a flow of sodium and calcium ions. The ion flow generates a neural signal. When it reaches its limit, the receptor goes into desensitisation mode. After reaching the limit, the receptor does not respond to any activity.

Thus, these subtypes manage the flow of important ions, which further regulates the neural signals. Our brain can only perform rationally when it has the right neural signals. Without them, it feels fuzzy.

Also, remember, nAChRs are present across several parts of your CNS. Hence, these subtypes don't influence just one region. For example, they also change neural connections in hippocampus, which is associated with learning and memory.

Lesson: The receptors might be tiny, but they are constantly shaping how we think, act, and remember. How?

MAINTAINING NEURAL CHEMISTRY

The receptors handle the quality and strength of the synapses. This function is very important since it helps filter out the weak synapses and make space to learn more. In absence of this process, the brain wont be able to adapt and learn new things. This process keeps the brain memory in check. The location of the subtype is important in this mechanism. If it is located at the nerve ending, it regulates the release of neurotransmitters (*presynaptic*). This activation maintains the release of chemicals like acetylcholine. In simple terms, the release of chemicals is the neural signal. Presynaptic shows that the subtypes are directly involved in neural communication.

When it is located at the receiving end of the synapse, it is known as *postsynaptic*. Once the subunit receives the signal, it opens the ion channels to allow ions into the cell. It shows that the message is received and is being acted upon! Thus, the subunits are responsible for both delivering and receiving the message as per their location.

But what happens when the subtypes don't function properly?

Disturbance in subtypes means disturbance in neural connections. When there is no proper communication in the brain, it means memory loss, difficulty in concentrating, and other psychological disorders like Schizophrenia and

Alzheimer's. It is important to learn about these disturbances to create better treatment policies. In tobacco-related diseases, we have been able to create effective medicines because of the right knowledge. Its understanding helps us understand which medication will work the best.

These tiny, minuscule particles, unknown to the naked eye, handle a bunch of important tasks. Thanks to these transmitters and their subtypes, we are able to learn, retain, act, and make decisions. Otherwise, it would have been pretty hard to work with a goldfish memory.

But, wait, can we actually observe and study receptors?

Well, yes, we can. Today, we stand at a point where, with the help of technology, we can analyse the receptors. Techniques like *X-ray crystallography* and *cryo-electron microscopy* have turned out to be landmark discoveries in research. They have provided important insights into ligand binding and ion channels. Using these techniques, one can see the change in synapses. This knowledge helps create right medicines. Medical experts are able to locate which substance can directly influence the receptors. So, how exactly does it work? Two simple technological advancements have accelerated the research field. The first is:

X-Ray Crystallography

This technique helps to see the atomic structure of a molecule. It basically tells location of every part. Let's take this through each step to understand the process better:

-Crystallization: It refers to aligning the molecules in order. This order helps to read the structure.

-X-Ray Diffraction: A beam of X-rays is aimed at a crystal. The X-ray is passed through it, which scatters the crystal.

-Diffraction pattern: The scattered rays produce an image. The process is known as diffraction. It is used to calculate a 3D structure.

-Electron Density Map: A 3D map helps to know where the electrons are located. This helps to know the atomic locations.

-Model Building: This is a detailed 3D model. It is the final structure that explains how the molecule works.

Cryo-Electron Microscopy

The second is Cryo-Electron Microscopy. It is a transmission electron microscope. Meaning? It allows us to look at molecules without crystallisation. It involves freezing them quickly and then observing with electrons. How does it happen?

-Vitrification: The molecules are frozen in liquid ethane till it freezes. This is performed instead of crystallisation. It is done to preserve the natural shape of the molecule.

-Electron Beam Imaging: This stage involves electrons to capture molecule images. It reveals finer details.

-Transmission Electron Microscopy: This is the name of the equipment used to transmit electrons to see images. It creates 2D images of the frozen molecules.

-Single Particle Analysis: Many images of the 2D molecules are captured. These are combined to form a 3D picture.

-3D Reconstruction: A 3D image helps to learn about the functioning of the molecule.

The images obtained have proved to be relevant. This has made it easier to understand addiction patterns and how to cope with them. Medical experts have been taking these studies seriously, primarily because the issue of nicotine addiction has been rising.

NICOTINE VS. PUBLIC HEALTH

We know that, in recent times, there has been a growing taste for nicotine. Hence, studies and development of techniques to understand the nicotine molecule are also important. We need to notice that outside the books, the issue of nicotine is very real and concerning. More and more youth are consuming nicotine in one way or another. Hence, for public health, it is important to focus on how we can extend sustainable healthcare.

Nicotine addiction has become a global issue. There are 1.3 billion active smokers around the world. It leads to 8 million deaths worldwide, along with 20 million cancers and respiratory cases. Young adults, as early as 10 years of age, are picking up the habit of smoking. World Health Organization is trying to tackle these challenges.

In the middle of all of this, technological progress in medicine helps us know where we stand and how we can help our youth.

It may surprise you to know that nicotine deaths directly affect the economy of the country. Every nation's government spends a huge budget on awareness campaigns, providing cost-friendly treatments. For instance, in 2018, the US spent 240 billion dollars on healthcare for smoking. It suffered a loss of 372 billion dollars in productivity because of nicotine related consequences. For India, we spend a total of 22.4 billion dollars on tobacco related healthcare. The cost of tobacco related death in monetary value is around 1324.5 billion rupees. This is in addition to the emotional burden it carries. Talking about it at a global level, tobacco healthcare expenditure comes down to 1.4 US trillion dollars, that is, 1,400,000,000,000! Not enough zeros to count on fingertips! The loss of productivity due to deaths has become a major issue that the government is taking stricter steps to address this issue.

We should also keep in mind that smokers are not welcome in most spaces. They are continuously looked down on. Importantly, it is smokers who are kept at a distance rather than smoking. It can cause people to develop an inferiority complex, further deepening their addiction. They develop a negative attitude and give up on cessation therapies. Hence, while we know it is an unhealthy habit, we should all show sympathy towards the victims of addiction. People across all age groups face this stigma. It is more for women and men with families. They are expected to follow a moral standard. Often, these people are not included in regular conversations, leading to isolation. Hence, to cope with loneliness, they feel pressed to hide behind nicotine.

The development and learning about the physiology of the human body is truly wonderful. It has given us the tools to work towards better health. Research is the key to discover a chance at better health. It will take global effort to resolve or reduce this health crisis. In this awareness spree, let's remember, we are against smoking, not the smoker!

Chapter – 12
TOWARDS A HEALTHY FUTURE

Reflection always helps people to break poor habits. As we move to the final section, it's good to wonder what more we can explore to handle nicotine addiction.

How can we make our future better?

Well, in a progressing world, it is not so surprising how times have changed. Half a century ago, people were not aware of the consequences of nicotine and companies were making big profits out of them. But today, thanks to the media and strict government policies, we have access to the right information about our health as consumers. We live in good times with good healthcare facilities. We can depend on progressive, tried and tested nicotine treatments. However, for the sake of our comfort, we often end up ignoring the process behind it.

Have you ever wondered about the process behind "test"?

While progress in medicine is always good news to humans, it takes toll on our surroundings. The same goes for nicotine treatments. Cessation medicines have been tested on both, animals and humans. Yes! You heard it right. As we benefit from the effective therapies, it won't be fair to ignore the cost, right?

Many animal welfare organisations have raised the issue of animal testing. There are serious consequences often ending in death. The debate over animal testing has been happening for a while. However, there has been no hopeful permanent solution.

ANSWERING THE LONG STANDING QUESTION

You may wonder, "*Why do people smoke when they know its side effects?*" People are not born as addicts. Yes, genes do play a role, but they do not define their addiction. People pick up habits as per their conditions. For example, people with mental disorders like anxiety and depression consume nicotine to feel happiness or for a "dopamine hit".

Similarly, people living in dismal conditions take nicotine as an escape route. Adolescents living in abusive environments look to substances to "feel better".

What is the way to go about helping these people ? Definitely not by labelling them. We need to identify the main factor that triggers addictive behaviour. An individual-based study can show us some light. It gives the promise of a healthy future.

But, How do we secure a healthy future?

An important question confronts us. How do we handle the growing use of nicotine among youth? At present, they have easy access to nicotine through cigarettes, vapes, e-cigarettes and other products. The wide availability of cigarettes does not help. Even as parents, we can't hold them at gunpoint and ask them not to not smoke. It's an independent choice.

What we *can* focus on is counselling and teaching them about the the health consequences.

As citizens, we do expect the policy makers to take effective steps. There has been increased global efforts, from funding, to treatments, to rehabilitation centres. But how much focus has been on the companies policies of organisations which are actually selling these products?

The tobacco industry is expanding. Ethical practices are the need of the hour. The government's duty is to ensure that tobacco companies follow the policies and inform their consumers of the possible health damage. Similarly, they should abide by ethical practices during testing. For testing, they should take approval from the Institutional Review Board or Ethics Committee.

This ensures that the product has been tested for:

- Risk to participants,
- Informed consent of the subject,
- Privacy and confidentiality, and
- Special consent for those who are mentally challenged, or disabled.

Different countries have adopted different models and go by different agencies and organisations' rules and recommendations. For example, the USA follows the Food and Drug Administration. It overlooks nicotine in NBT products like e-cigarettes or patches. The nicotine levels should comply with Good Clinical Practice. Europe follows the European Medicines Agency. It looks after the nicotine therapists and clinical research.

There are guidelines from international organisations like Framework Convention on Tobacco Control and World Health Organisation. They have laid out public health guidelines, and ethical guidelines for nicotine consumption and research.

Can we take over the MNCs?

We are aware that companies including the tobacco industry are profit oriented. But it does not mean they can blindly exploit their customers. As part of their Corporate Social Responsibility, they need to ensure they do not hurt the well being of the human community. What are these responsibilities?

- Right information to consumers,
- Fair independent reviews,
- Disclosure of their interests,
- Any health concerns.

The companies should also provide guidelines about right dosage and safe use. They need to address waste management techniques. Remember, meeting this requirement is very important, if we want to live in a healthy environment.

But what if they don't?

It is not new news. Many times big MNCs have taken the liberty to increase profits by sidelining standard practices. They have been given warnings, asked to pay fines, and change their working methods. Some times it led to good results, whereas at other times, things remined as they were.

THE NECESSITY OF TOBACCO INDUSTRY

The tobacco industry provides employment to thousands. Abolishing it is not the solution. Hence, governments have been taking a different approach, a more liberal one. There is an aim to reach for a balance.

For our future generations' health, we must focus on awareness campaigns and therapies. The authorities can bring strict laws for age restrictions. Also, we need to end the stigma associated with the person and start addressing the habit of "*smoking*". Basically when we smoke cigarettes, we are consuming the final product. The product is manufactured by companies. Hence, there are ethical concerns involved at every level.

- The companies should not benefit at the cost of the health of its consumers.
- The research units should not cause animal abuse.
- The government should have policies which promote public health.
- And as civilians, we should promote awareness campaigns.

With combined efforts, we can have healthy citizens and strong national health.

Let's see what the new research has to offer.

Talking from the grounds, there are many factors which directly affect policy making. It is important to follow epidemiology which is the science of studying public health across populations. It helps to study health patterns, causes, and effects in different populations. With the help of this science, we can analyse the risks and preventative measures when it comes to nicotine.

How so?

Let me explain:

Region: It is generally seen that individuals from lower-income groups and rural places rely on nicotine. There are reasons for it. They are not aware of the massive consequences. It is the most affordable and easily accessible coping tool. Also, they don't have access to cessation therapies.

Gender: Males tend to start early and smoke more. In metro and urban areas the gender gap is reducing. But typically, males smoke more and take to addiction.

Age: Smoking generally starts around 13-15 years of age. It reaches the addiction stage around 18-20 years. Awareness programs and counselling at this age can prevent long term addiction.

Medium of Use: Traditional uses of tobacco are declining. Today, we see a rise in e-cigarettes, and smokeless tobacco in teenagers. Despite this change, cigarettes continue to be widely used across all ages.

A DIFFERENT INSIGHT

These are scientific public studies. Similarly we have *Longitudinal Studies.* They track the nicotine use over a longer period of time and include the above-mentioned factors like age, region, gender. A popular longitudinal study conducted is known as PATH study or **Population Assessment of Tobacco and Health study.** This was conducted across different regions of the USA to study tobacco behaviour and find suitable solutions. It revealed interesting insights:

- People liked to smoke flavoured products more and frequently.
- It showed the surroundings and mental health and its influence on smoking patterns,
- Youth today uses e-cigarettes more.

If it's getting too vague, let's understand it with an example. A case study will help to understand how various factors influence addiction pattern. Aryan, a 16 year old male from a privileged economic background started vaping e-cigarettes. He developed a habit under the influence of friends/social pressure. From occasional puffs to using nicotine regularly, Aryan started vaping to feel the "dopamine hit". It eventually lead to dependence.

His friend Akash also started smoking with him and developed dependence. Akash came from a vulnerable economic position and did not have as many resources as Aryan. Because of his better socioeconomic position, Aryan got the needed therapy to quit. He attended CBT, had support from his parents, and the means to carry on cessation therapies. However Akash didn't have the means to receive the same support.

Result?

Akash developed extreme cravings, anger issues, and irritation when he couldn't have nicotine. Addiction impacted his physical and mental health. It created issues in his personal life, rifts with his family, and directly affected his health. Because of his addiction, he faced biased behaviour from his neighbours. This pushed him into isolation and further depression. The case of Aryan and Akash shows clearly that nicotine use has influenced many people. Some were able to come out of the trap, but most couldn't.

But, the situation is not hopeless.

Despite challenges, there are efforts to fight nicotine addiction. If there are sad affairs, there are inspiring stories too. No effort made towards quitting goes waste. Lakhs of people quit on time because they know of the damages, thanks to the awareness campaigns. Several other thousands receive treatment on time, thanks to the therapies, and many receive the needed emotional support thanks to help groups.

As I end this book, I repeat, the fight is not against **smokers**, but the habit of **smoking**.

It is not about just breaking a habit. Its rediscovering strength, will power, and health. It's a step to live freely where no addiction leads you. You are your own sailor. Everyday of your quitting journey is a reminder towards a healthy life, a guilt free life.

Quit nicotine and start the beginning of a **HEALTHY** and **HAPPY** life!

END